DENGUE

Prevention & Control

THE LAHORE MODEL OF SUCCESS

KHALID SHERDIL

FARAN NARU

AHMAD RAJWANA

Copyright © 2012 by Khalid Sherdil
ISBN-13: 978-1478225454
ISBN-10: 1478225459

DEDICATIONS

This book is dedicated to the Government officials who sacrificed their own life, health and well-being to prevent and cure the Dengue fever in Lahore. This includes doctors, nurses, and the spraying staff, that went beyond their call of duty and relentlessly served others while endangering their own lives by exposing themselves to the vector.

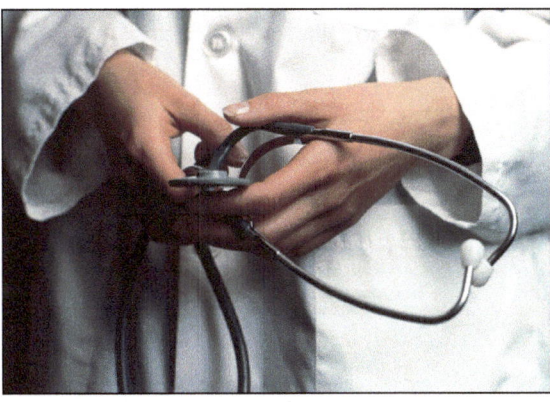

ACKNOWLEDGEMENTS

Provincial Disaster Management Authority obtained the information provided by all relevant departments of the Government of Punjab, Pakistan. All of the information was provided under the guidance of these Departments' Secretaries, Director Generals and other related staff. The Department Heads have created great examples of epidemic control and through this book their productive experience can be communicated to tropical and other states that continue to face the threat of Dengue outbreak.

The authors of this book acknowledge the substantial contributions made by the following persons and express their gratitude to them:

- Mr. Muhammad Jahanzaib Khan — Secretary, Health Department
- Mr. Mohyuddin Ahmed Wani — Secretary, Information Department
- Mr. Arif Nadeem — Secretary, Agriculture Department
- Mr. Javed Akhtar — Secretary, Social Welfare Department
- Mr. Syed Mubbashir Raza — Secretary, Implementation and Coordination Department
- Mr. Muhammad Irfan Elahi — Secretary, Irrigation Department
- Mr. Sajjad Saleem Hotiana — Secretary, Environment Department
- Mr. Sohail Aamir — Secretary, HUD & PHE Department
- Mr. Khizer Hayat Gondal — Secretary, Local Government Department
- Mr. Muhammad Aslam Kamboh — Secretary, Schools Education Department
- Dr. Ejaz Munir — Secretary, Higher Education Department
- Mr. Tariq Mahmood Pasha — Secretary, Auqaf Department
- Mr. Shahnawaz Badr — Secretary, Forests Department
- Mr. Hassan Iqbal — Secretary, Labour and Human Resource Department
- Mr. Khalid Masood Chaudhry — Secretary, Cooperatives Department
- Mr. Muhammad Yusuf — Secretary, Transport Department
- Mr. Jawad Rafiq Malik — Commissioner, Lahore
- Mr. Dawood Bareach — Special Secretary, Health Department
- Mr. Ahad Khan Cheema — District Coordination Officer, Lahore
- Mr. Mujahid Sherdil — Director General, PDMA, Punjab
- Mr. Shehryar Sultan — Director General, Local Government Department
- Mr. Abdul Jabbar Shaheen — Director General, PHA & LDA
- Mr. Anjum Ali — Director General, Agriculture (Ext) Department
- Dr. Muhammad Aslam Chaudhry — Director General, Director General Health Services
- Dr. Muhammad Anwar Janjua — MIS Director, Director General Health Services
- Mr. Farooq Ahmad — Computer Program Officer, Directorate General Health
- Mr. Azmat Ali Awan — GIS Specialist, iMMAP
- Mr. Mohammad Jarjaish Hussain — Information Management Officer / GIS Specialist, IMMAP
- Mr. Omer Younus — Information Management Officer / GIS Specialist, IMMAP
- Dr. M Akram Arain — Deputy District Officer, Health Department, Samnabad
- Mr. Sher Alam Mehsud — Vice Commissioner, PESSI
- Mr. Khalid Majeed — GM Operations, Solid Waste Management Company
- Mr. Zaman Narejo — Director, PDMA, Punjab
- Mr. Nisar Ahmed Sani — Assistant Director, PDMA, Punjab

TABLE OF CONTENTS

LIST OF FIGURES

LIST OF TABLES

ACRONYMS

Abbreviation	Expansion
CBC	Complete Blood Count
CDGL	City District Government, Lahore
CERC	Central Emergency Response Committee
DCO	District Coordination Officer
DG	Director General
DGHS	Directorate General Health Services
DHA	Defence Housing Authority
DHQ	District Headquarter Hospital
ECRS	Electronic Complaint Routing System
EDO	Executive District Officer
EDO (H)	Executive District Officer (Health)
EPA	Environmental Protection Agencey
GIS	Geographic Information System
IRS	Internal Residual Spray
LDA	Lahore Development Authority
LG&CD	Local Government and Community Development
LWMC	Lahore Waste Management Company
MNA	Member of National Assembly
MPA	Member of Provincial Assembly
NGO	Non-Government Organization
OPD	Outdoor Patient Department
PDMA	Provincial Disaster Management Authority
PDMC	Punjab Dental and Medical Commission
PHA	Parks and Horticulture Authority
PITB	Punjab Information Technology Board
RHC	Rural Health Centre
SMS	Short Messaging Service
SOP	Standard Operating Procedure
THH	Tehsil Headquarter Hospital
TMA	Town Municipal Administration
TMO	Town Municipal Officer
UC	Union Council
WASA	Water and Sanitation Agency
WHO	World Health Organization

FOREWORD

Muhammad Shahbaz Sharif
Chief Minister, Punjab

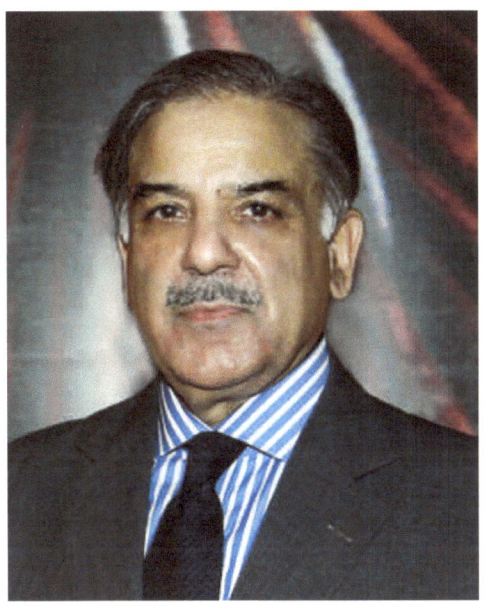

I wish to dedicate this book to the brave, generous and resilient people of Lahore, and of Punjab, who fought valiantly with the menace of dengue fever, for the service of humanity.

As one of the active participants of the anti-dengue campaign, it was my honour to witness the services of all the doctors, nurses, paramedics, sanitary staff, medical students, Post Graduate (PG) trainees, pharmacists, specialists, scientists, hospital staff, entomologists, IT experts, politicians, social activists and ordinary citizens, who joined hands with the Government of the Punjab to make our efforts in curbing the epidemic, a success. I wish to recognize and appreciate their heroic efforts.

Dengue is a phenomenon that cannot be eradicated permanently. It is in the essence of the times that we develop a long term strategy to control it in Punjab. I would request all the people who were with me in this effort, either directly or indirectly, to adopt well thought-out and integrated strategies to combat this menace. Our success depends on and will be evaluated during the coming season.

I hope and pray that we are able to serve our nation and save the lives of our fellow brothers and sisters for the collective benefit of humanity.

FOREWORD

Nasir Mahmood Khosa
Chief Secretary, Punjab

Punjab province faced a massive outbreak of Dengue fever in the fall of 2011. All the Government Departments responded to this epidemic, and contributed in the vector control efforts which is commendable.

I wish to avail this opportunity to thank all of our staff for their diligence and perseverance. Our staff has shown an unshakable resolve in responding to the Dengue epidemic. All the Government Departments prepared their policy recommendations, shared the responsibility and delivered in whatever role they were engaged. These recommendations were accordingly enacted with a commitment and dedication that was desirous of the Government at a time when the Dengue fever was rapidly spreading across the city of Lahore. Rapid spread of Dengue fever was noticed in the Urban Centers in Lahore after the monsoon downpours. All the departments utilized their relevant expertise to streamline the efforts. The Punjab Government responded with a well-coordinated plan to eliminate the source of Dengue fever, and to check the further spread of this disease.

The City District Government, Lahore, along with the Health, Agriculture, PHA, LDA, LG&CD, Transport, Schools, Environment and other Departments conducted chemical control including larvicidal activity, fumigation, and fogging in all Union Councils, Parks, Graveyards, Bus Stands and Tyre Shops respectively. The Fisheries Department was deputed to conduct biological control of vector. Health Department improved the health care facilities in hospitals operational in both public and private sectors. High Dependency Units (HDUs) were established at all the Tertiary Care (Teaching) as well as Secondary Care (DHQ) level Hospitals for the better management of Dengue fever patients.

A massive awareness campaign was launched with the support of all allied Departments which contributed in control of Dengue Fever Epidemic. The establishment of Central Emergency Response Committee (CERC) and Town Emergency Response Teams (TERTs) was an innovation which provided the direction at operational level all along.

I hope that this high level of inter-sectoral coordination and integrated efforts will serve as a model to control any such epidemic in future.

PREFACE

Khalid Sherdil
Former Director General, PDMA

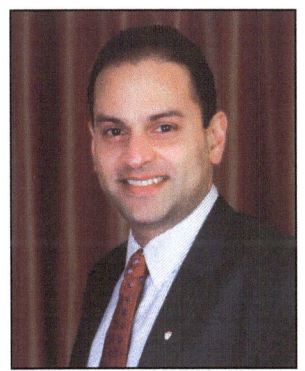

Our daily routines started at 5:30 am. The Dining Hall of 180-H Model Town, Lahore, which is the Chief Minister's Camp Office, was converted into a War Room. Every morning at 6:45 am, government officers gathered at the War Room, carrying Digital Proofs of the progress of past 24 hours. At 7:00 am, the brain storming session commenced, where elected representatives, officers, journalists, international advisors, scientists, NGO representatives, technocrats, and other members of society presented their work, exchanged ideas, received feedback, faced constructive criticism, and in the end came up with a course of action for the next 24 hours. Meeting terminated by 9 am, so that the officers could be back in their offices to implement the planned strategy.

It was this tireless effort, which brought a 300% decrease in the Dengue casualty rate, as is statistically demonstrated in this book. There was no holiday, not even Sunday, because there could be no rest when the public was under threat. The meetings were chaired by the Chief Minister, Mohammad Shahbaz Sharif. Leading from the front has always been his habit, as was proven during the Super Floods of 2010, Pakistan's worst ever disaster. And now this epidemic was turning out to be another disaster, but this time it was striking the *Heart of Pakistan*, Lahore.

The war room ritual commenced with the Health Secretary giving an initial overview, followed by a round-robin brief from each departmental head. Each briefing had to be complemented with digital proofs, i.e., time-stamped photographs of last 24 hours' action. These were then geo-positioned onto satellite imagery, so as to get a visual picture in a Geographical Information System (sample maps are shown in this book). In this way, through a scientific approach, the battle was launched against the mosquito.

International advisors from Sri Lanka were first to arrive, followed by the Indonesians. These countries have tropical-cum-equatorial climates, most conducive to Dengue. They informed us that it would be a long fought war, lasting 30 years in Sri Lanka, with thousands of casualties. But at the end of the year, they were amazed at the speed with which the Punjab Govt. had responded, and the steepness of our learning curve, which resulted in an all out assault on the virus, nipping it in the bud by deploying 30 years of acquired knowledge in a period of three months.

What were the reasons behind the success of this Lahore model? How were the casualties confined to 21,292 patients with 352 deaths whereas historic data was predicting 55,000 patients (with 900 deaths)? Can this model be replicated in other countries? This book attempts to describe the Lahore model, and shows that it indeed can be replicated at a fast pace in any other region, using an integrated and holistic approach where each Government Department utilizes its maximum potential, in a more coordinated fashion. Indeed, the Lahore Model is itself a replication of other best practices from Sri Lanka, Indonesian and other countries, though at an accelerated supersonic pace. The objective behind this book is to impart our acquired knowledge to others, so as to save lives in other parts of the world where Dengue or other Mosquito vector diseases strike. We hope this text is circulated in libraries as a primary and original data-cum-narrative for reference in future research in fields of Public Health, Public Administration and Clinical studies.

The objective of this book is to articulate the best practices undertaken by the Departments of the Government of Punjab and propose similar guidelines for developing an Integrated Dengue Control Program so that other administrators may use the experiences of Lahore Model to prevent dengue in their domains. The guidelines are developed in the light of the productive experiences of Government Departments of the Punjab. Apart from Lahore, Dengue also spread to other Districts such as Faisalabad, Rawalpindi, Multan, Sheikhupura, Okara, Rahim Yar Khan and Pakpattan. Although the incidence of this disease is considerably low in these districts, the district administrators in these areas can certainly use the guidelines and experiences to control this disease before it affects a larger percentage of the population. Administrators may engage the representatives of different departments to form and implement a holistic control program.

Roles and Responsibilities

Almost all Government Departments contributed in the vector control efforts in Lahore. These departments utilized their relevant expertise to streamline the efforts. These departments shared the responsibility and delivered in whatever role they were engaged in. The Agriculture Department created a team of entomologists to study the prevalence of larvae and adult mosquitoes. The Auqaf Department engaged religious scholars and madaris in public awareness campaigns. The Cooperatives Department initiated a comprehensive cleanliness drive with the help of different housing societies of Lahore. The Environment Department conducted a tyre management campaign. The Forests and Fisheries Department planned and implemented a biological control program utilizing the fish that feed on larvae. The Health Department collected data from all health facilities to advise the required changes to the vector control program.

The Higher Education Department conducted an awareness campaign with the help of college students. Lahore Waste Management Company launched an aggressive campaign for cleanliness and removal of garbage. The Local Government Department conducted fumigation of different graveyards. Parks and Horticulture Authority conducted the fumigation of all parks of Lahore. The Services and General Administration Department worked on the removal of debris from government offices. The School Education Department initiated a school cleanliness drive in which the schools were cleaned, fumigated and inspected. The Social Welfare Department mobilized NGOs to provide healthcare services to a large number of patients with Dengue related symptoms. The Transport Department cleaned and fumigated different bus stands of Lahore. The City District Government, Lahore conducted fogging, internal residual sprays and larvicidal activities across the city.

The above mentioned efforts serve as an example for administrators world over, who may face a similar challenge. Based on the experiences of the various departments of Punjab, specific interventions are suggested for each sector at the end of each chapter delineating that department's efforts. The Dengue prevention and control was an integrated multi-department effort. Hence this book devotes a chapter to each department.

Sample of public awareness material   Fig. 1

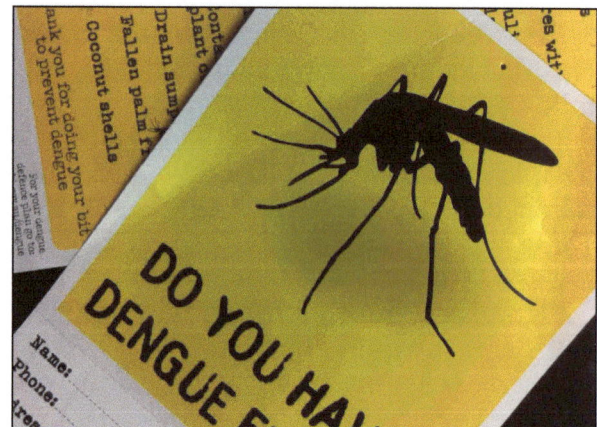

Punjab province inhabits more than 100 million people making it larger than any European country. The Dengue fever epidemic in the Fall of 2011 affected more that 21,000 people of Punjab. Urban centers in Lahore saw a rapid spread of Dengue fever after the monsoon downpours. More than 18,000 cases of this fever were reported from the city of Lahore. Although most of these patients recovered, the fever led to 352 deaths. About 85% of the total cases were reported in Lahore alone. The Government responded by eliminating the source of this fever, and by checking further spread of the disease.

A street after monsoon rain   Fig. 2

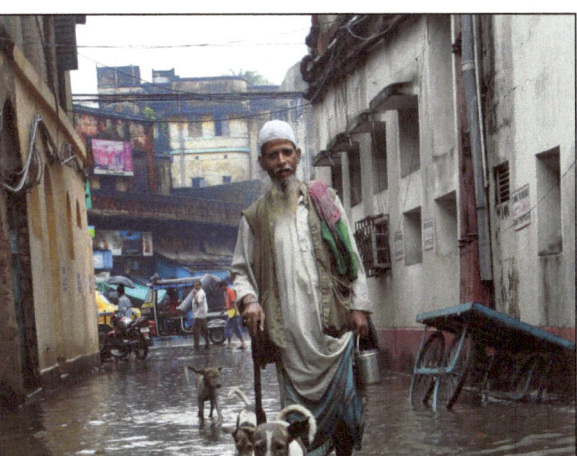

Geographic location of Punjab   Fig. 3

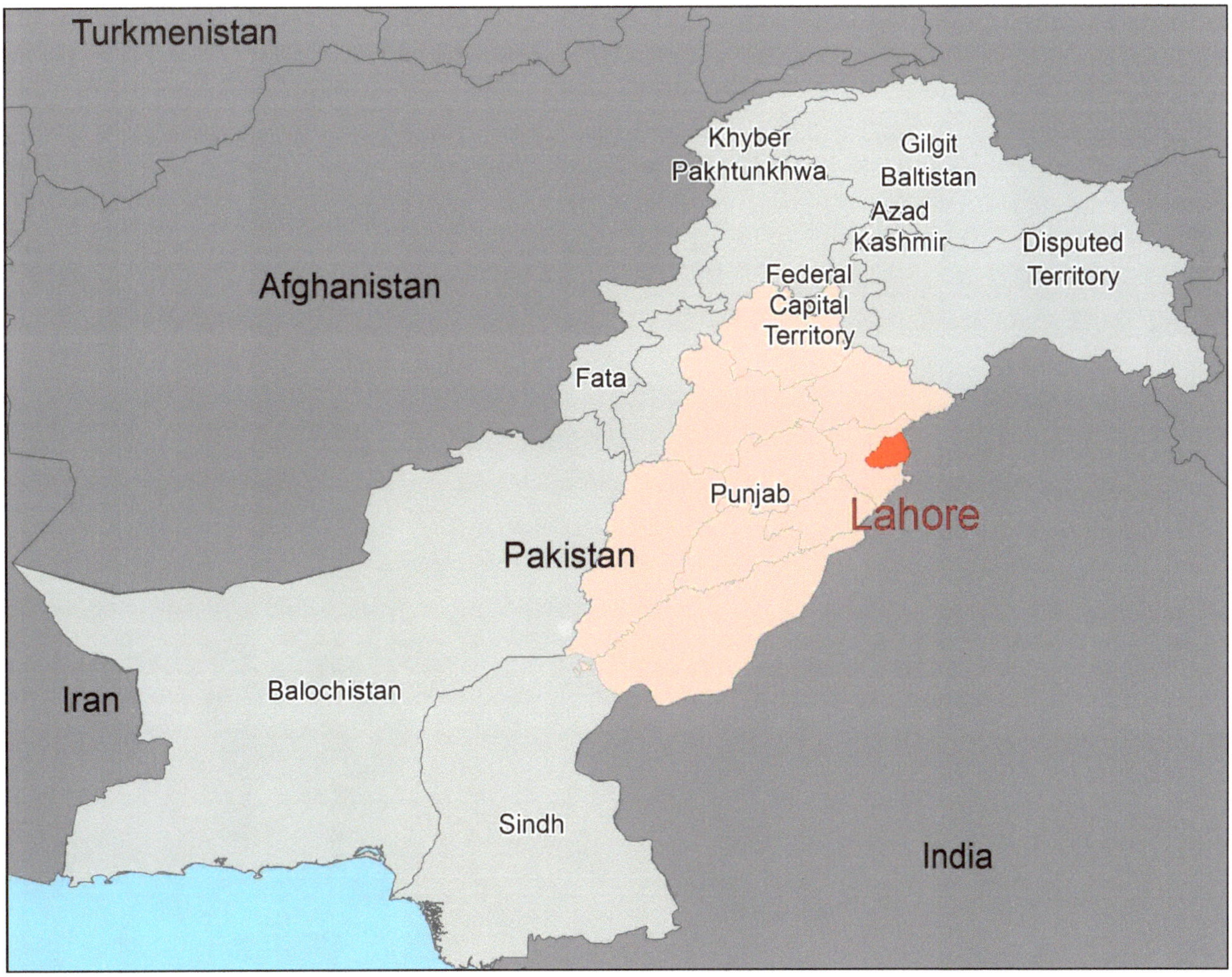

Turkmenistan

Afghanistan

Khyber
Pakhtunkhwa

Gilgit
Baltistan

Azad
Kashmir

Disputed
Territory

Federal
Capital
Territory

Fata

Punjab

Lahore

Pakistan

Iran

Balochistan

Sindh

India

The higher cadres of the government strategized a vector control program and its implementation was devolved to the various governmental departments. The various departments then divided their responsibilities and coordinated with each other to ensure the gradual elimination of Dengue fever. Their coordination serves as an example for an Integrated Dengue Control Program that can be adopted by any area facing this epidemic.

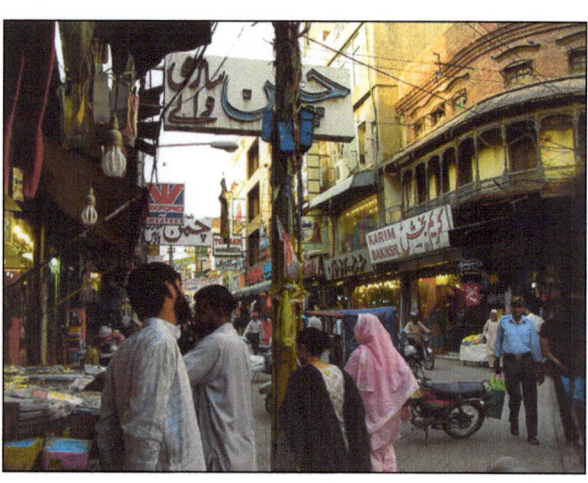

Anarkali Bazzar, Data Gunj Bakhash Town *Fig. 4*

Geographic location of Lahore *Fig. 5*

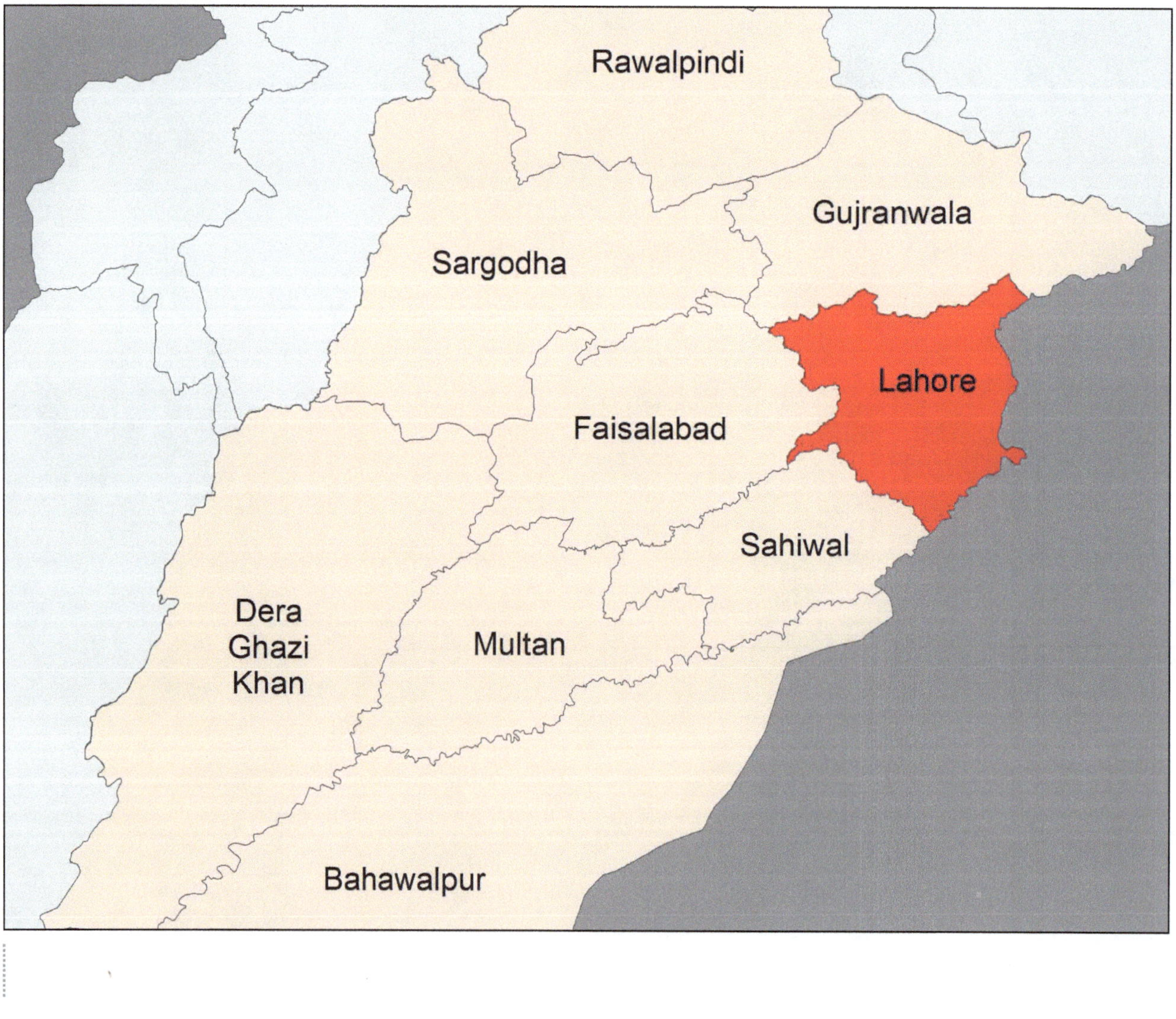

Rawalpindi

Gujranwala

Sargodha

Lahore

Faisalabad

Sahiwal

Dera Ghazi Khan

Multan

Bahawalpur

Dengue is a vector-borne disease caused by the transmission of flavivirus through mosquitoes such as *Aedes Aegyptus* or *Aedes Albopictus*. A large proportion of the world's population lives in over a hundred countries where Dengue is in an endemic state. The epidemic outbreak of this disease can have devastating consequences. More than 350 persons lost their lives due to the outbreak of Dengue in Pakistan. The World Health Organization (WHO) estimates that 50 million cases of Dengue occur every year. Figure 7 highlights the countries that are at a risk of on going transmission of Dengue fever. Apart from Pakistan, this disease has affected a number of other tropical countries such as Indonesia, Srilanka, Brazil and India.

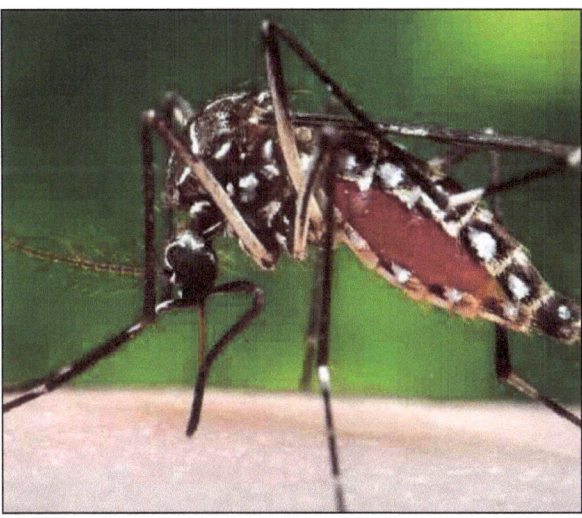

Aedes Mosquitoe — Fig. 6

Centers for Disease Control and Prevention. (n.d.). Dengue Map: A CDC-Health Map Collaboration. Retrieved March 01, 2012, from Health Map: http://www.healthmap.org/dengue/index.php

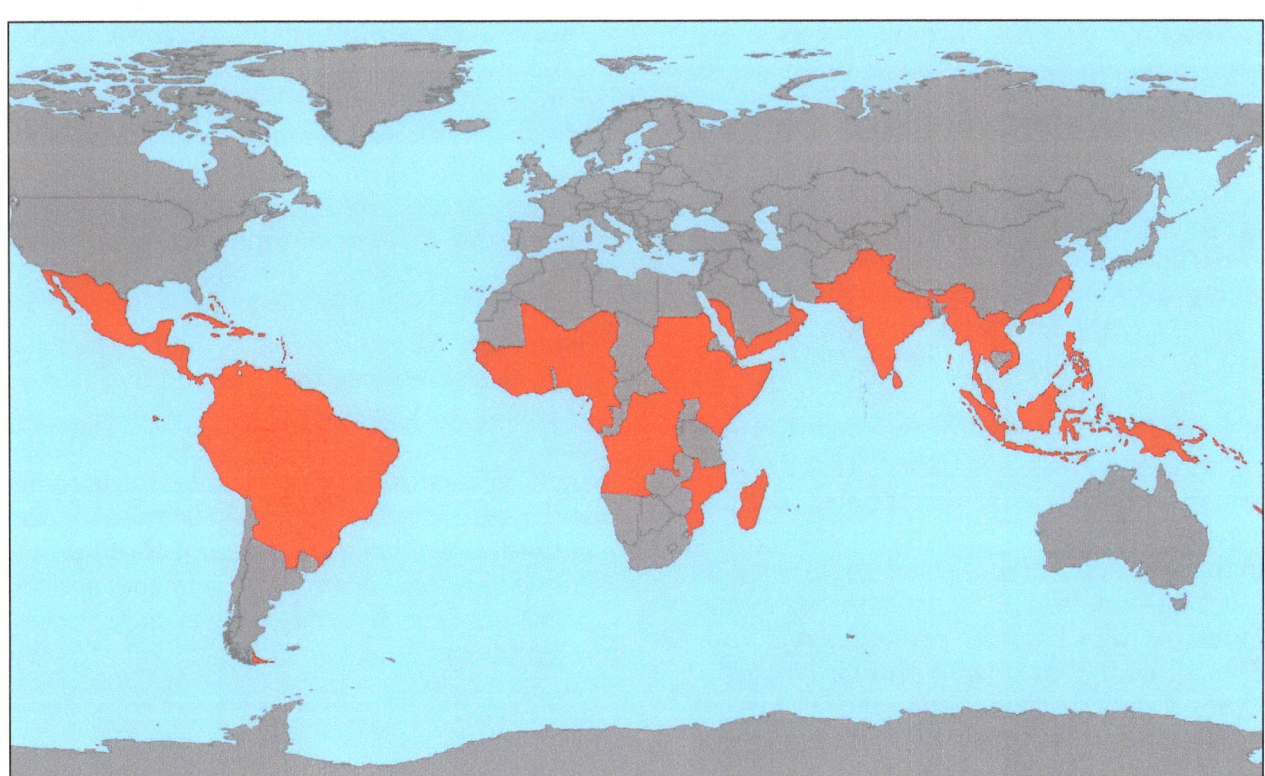

Dengue risk areas — Fig. 7

EPIDEMIC RESEARCH ON THE GEOGRAPHIC SPREAD OF DENGUE FEVER

The Provincial Disaster Management Authority (PDMA), Punjab, undertook a holistic research to understand the reasons that led to the rapid outbreak of the Dengue epidemic. The purpose of the research was to understand the core problems that contributed to the spread of this disease and to propose solutions to eliminate these problems in coming years before the epidemic sprouts again.

Hypotheses

The research was undertaken to test the validity of the following two hypotheses:

1. Ideal habitats such as Parks and Graveyards encouraged widespread breeding of the vector and thus the increased mosquito population infected a greater number of people in Lahore.

2. The high population density of Lahore contributed to the rapid spread of this fever.

Results

PDMA observed that the highest number of patients resided in areas that were close to Parks and Graveyards. Lahore is administratively divided into 150 Union Councils. Lahore's worst affected Union Council was Model Town followed by Race Course and Mozang. The Model Town area contains Model Town Park, the Race Course Union Council is home to Lahore's largest Parks: Bagh-e-Jinnah and Jillani Park. Mozang area contains Miani Sahib, one of the largest Graveyards in the world. All of these landmarks acted as ideal habitats for *Aedes* mosquitoes as the monsoon rains left fresh water in small puddles all over these Parks and Graveyards. Union Councils containing Lahore's largest Parks and Graveyards generated the highest number of patients.

This proved PDMA's first hypothesis that ideal habitats increased the vector population which led to a greater number of patients in the areas surrounding their habitats. PDMA reached this conclusion by GIS mapping of the data of Dengue cases provided by Health Department.

The second hypothesis of PDMA was rejected. Model Town has considerably less population density compared to inner city of Lahore. More than 330 patients from Model Town had reported Dengue fever till 30th September 2011. On the other hand the Androon Texali Gate is one of the most densely populated areas of Lahore but only 19 patients from this areas reported Dengue fever till the end of September 2011.

The Government of Punjab was well aware that Parks and Graveyards acted as ideal habitats for *Aedes* mosquitoes in the post-monsoon season and so it initiated a comprehensive chemical control program in these places.

Parks and Horticulture Authority (PHA) conducted fogging in all the major Parks of Lahore, while the Local Government and Community Development Department conducted fogging in all the major Graveyards of the city. These chemical control activities significantly decreased the vector population in these areas. The Agriculture Department mobilized a team of Entomologists that studied the presence of vector in all areas of Lahore. This study took place from 20th September 2011 to late October 2011. The data from this study was also mapped by PDMA. The map of vector presence revealed low presence of mosquitoes in areas with Parks and Graveyards immediatleyafter the fogging and vector control. That map is an evidence of the success that the Government of Punjab has achieved in controlling the further spread of Dengue fever by eradicating vector colonies in Parks and Graveyards.

Methodology

The PDMA conducted individual analyses of each town. The purpose was to identify the areas which were generating the highest number of Dengue patients. The map for each town was analyzed and aggregated in the comprehensive map of Lahore. The comprehensive map of Dengue cases was juxtaposed with the map of vector prevalence. The comparison of these two maps highlighted the areas that were the highest priority for chemical control because of the presence of adult mosquitoes or larvae in those areas even after the chemical control.

The Health Department collected data on Dengue patients from hospitals across Punjab. Most of the Dengue patients provided their home addresses or neighbourhood information. Those addresses were mapped to the level of Union Councils where they resided. This exercise was conducted by all the Town Municipal Administrations (TMA) of Lahore. In this way, PDMA was able to determine the locations of most of the Dengue patients with the help of the Health department and the TMAs. The information on Union Councils was then streamlined to identify the Union Councils where the greatest number of Dengue patients resided.

Apart from this study, PDMA also mapped the areas that had a high prevalence of *Aedes* mosquitoes. The Agriculture Department mobilized 70 Entomologists to conduct more than 12,000 spot-checks identifying areas that had larvae or adult mosquitoes' presence. The percentage of hotspots in each Union Council was mapped to identify Union Councils where there might have been higher population levels of Mosquitoes.

The visual representation of this data on GIS was used to analyze if the chemical control undertaken by the government of Punjab had an impact on vector prevalence.

Data Collection Process *Fig. 8*

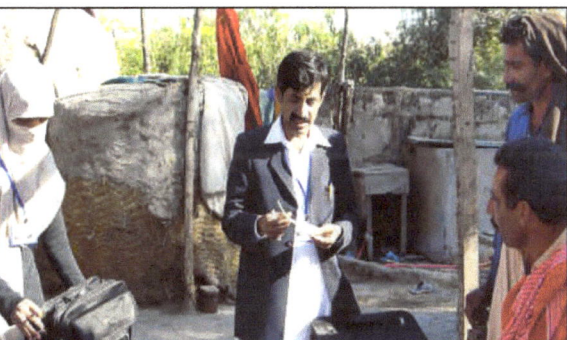

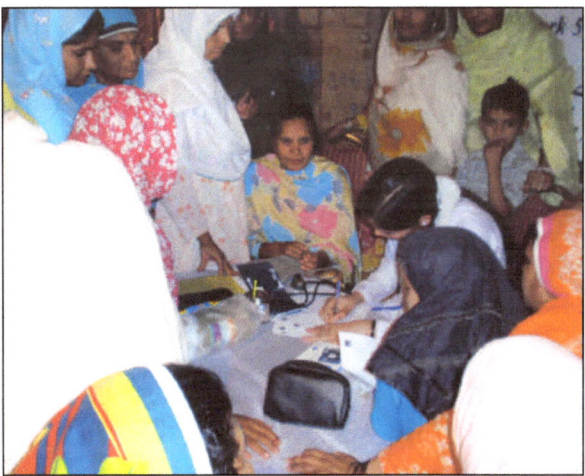

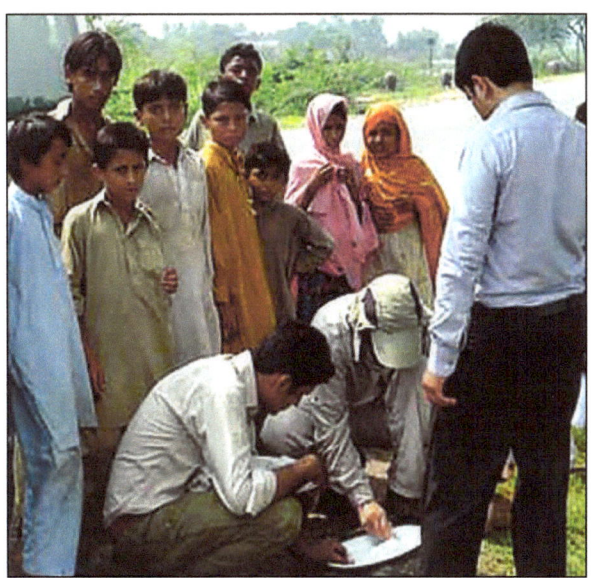

Figure 9 shows the map of distribution of patients across Lahore.

Lahore is administratively divided into nine towns and a cantonement region . The towns are then further divided into Union Councils (UCs). Union Council is the smallest administrative area in Pakistan and the city of Lahore comprises 150 Union Councils. PDMA studied the addresses of 11,000 patients to map the Towns and Union Councils where they resided. After a lengthy exercise, it was revealed that most of the Dengue patients resided in Data Gunj Buksh, Gulberg and Cantonment areas. Towns such as Aziz Bhatti and Wahga were the least affected areas.

Town wise summary of Dengue fever cases

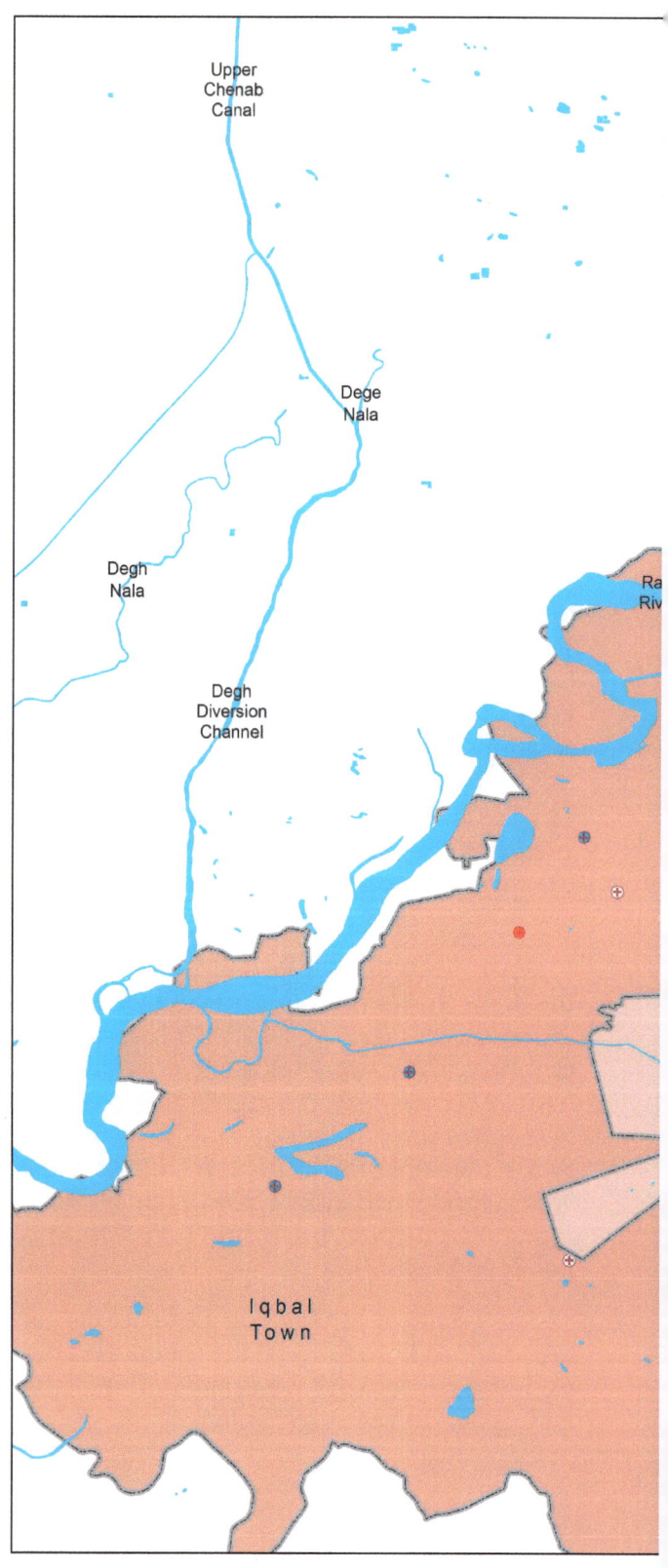

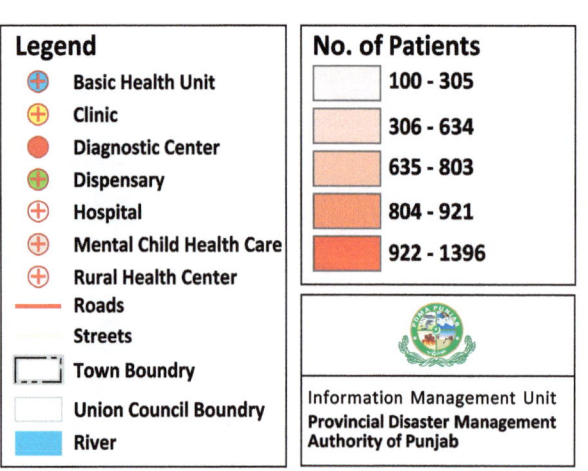

Legend

	Basic Health Unit
	Clinic
	Diagnostic Center
	Dispensary
	Hospital
	Mental Child Health Care
	Rural Health Center
	Roads
	Streets
	Town Boundry
	Union Council Boundry
	River

No. of Patients

	100 - 305
	306 - 634
	635 - 803
	804 - 921
	922 - 1396

Information Management Unit
Provincial Disaster Management Authority of Punjab

as of Sept. 30, 2011

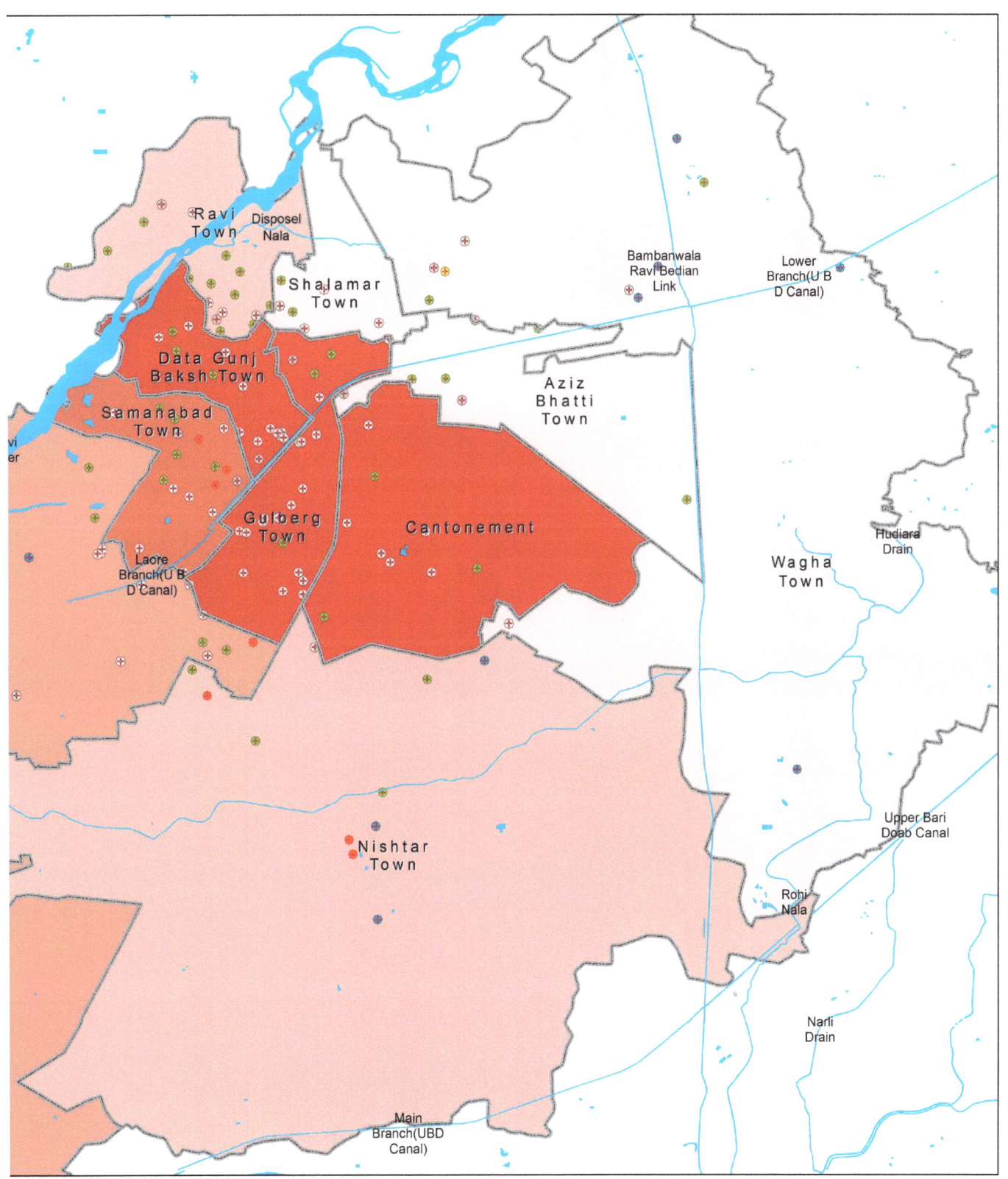

Aziz Bhatti Town

Mughalpura is the worst affected Union Council in Aziz Bhatti Town. More than 60 patients had reported Dengue fever from this Union Council till the end of September 2011. Compared to other towns of Lahore, Aziz Bhatti is one of the least affected areas. However the Mughalpura Union Council borders Data Gunj Buksh Town, which is one of the worst affected towns of Lahore. Shalimar Garden, a centuries old park, might have acted as a potential habitat of *Aedes* mosquitoes in this area but that cannot be established with certainty.

Figure 10 shows the map of geographic distribution of the patients of Dengue fever who residing in Aziz Bhatti Town.

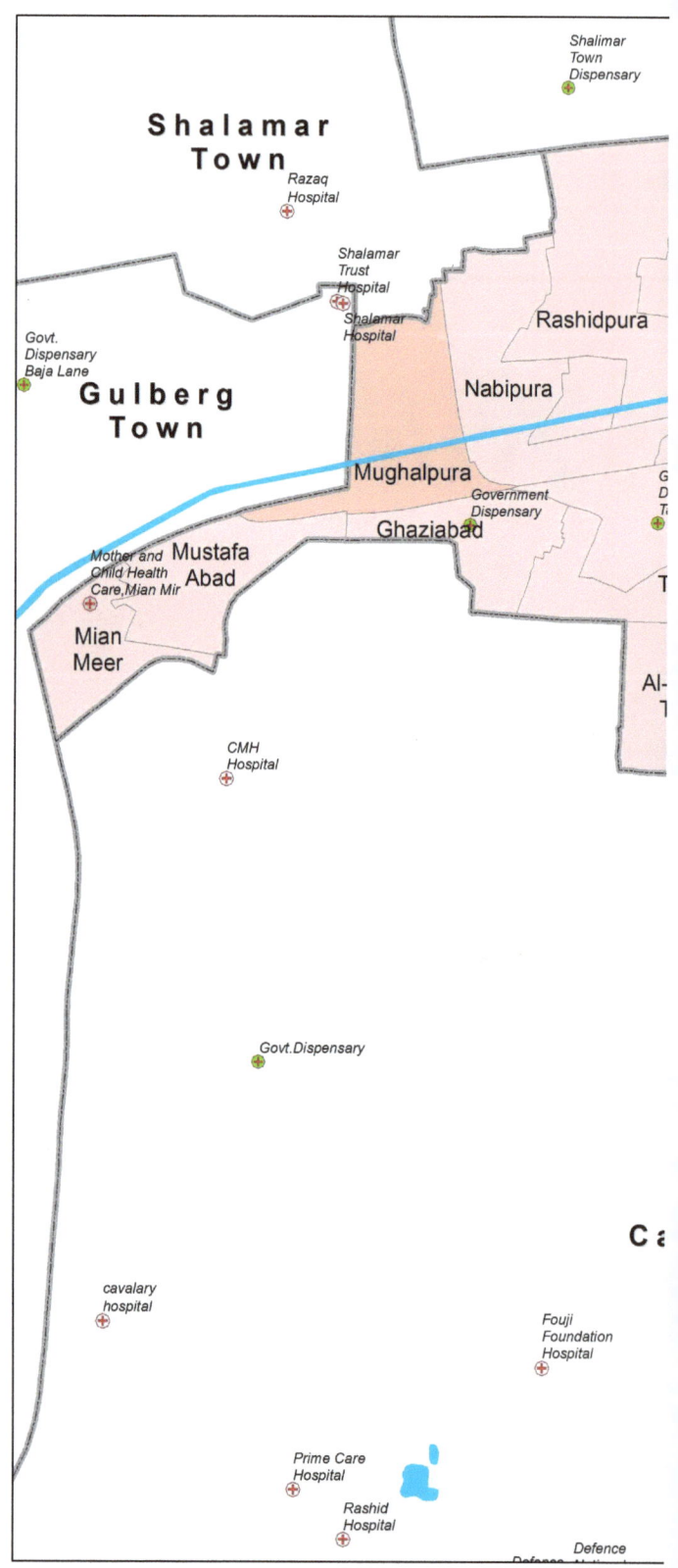

Aziz Bhatti Town: Union Council wise summ

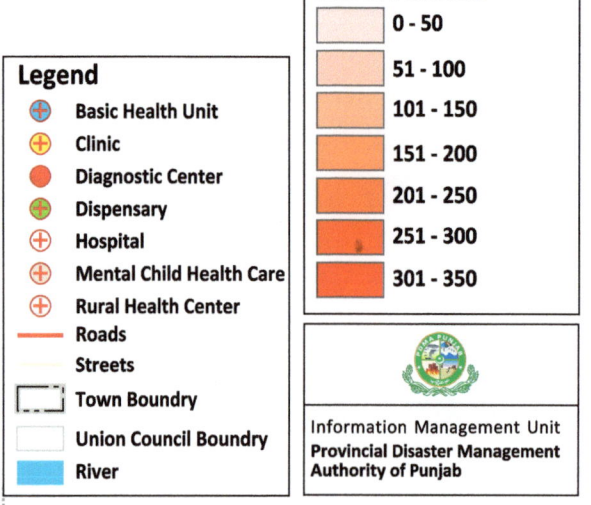

Legend	
⊕	Basic Health Unit
⊕	Clinic
●	Diagnostic Center
⊕	Dispensary
⊕	Hospital
⊕	Mental Child Health Care
⊕	Rural Health Center
—	Roads
	Streets
▭	Town Boundry
▭	Union Council Boundry
▬	River

No. of Patients

	0 - 50
	51 - 100
	101 - 150
	151 - 200
	201 - 250
	251 - 300
	301 - 350

Information Management Unit
Provincial Disaster Management Authority of Punjab

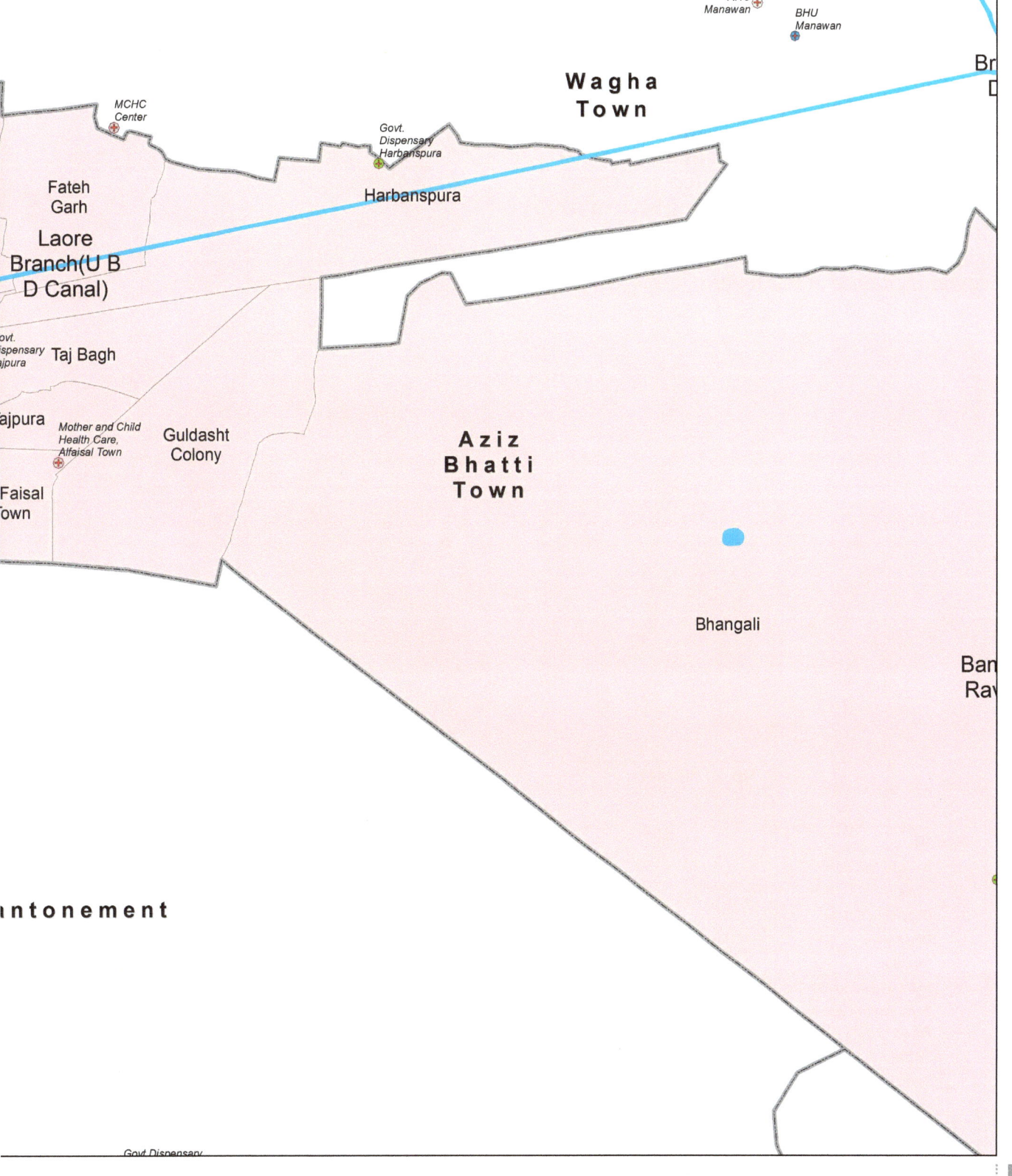

Nishtar Town

Nishtar Town was not as severely affected, but its northern part did witness a substantial Dengue related activity. The Ismail Nagar area containing Lahore General Hospital was the worst affected Union Council of Nishtar Town. More than 88 patients residing in this area were diagnosed with Dengue fever by the end of September 2011. More than 300 Dengue patients were admitted at General Hospital at any given date during September and October 2011. The southern Union Councils have a lower population density and lower incidence of this fever.

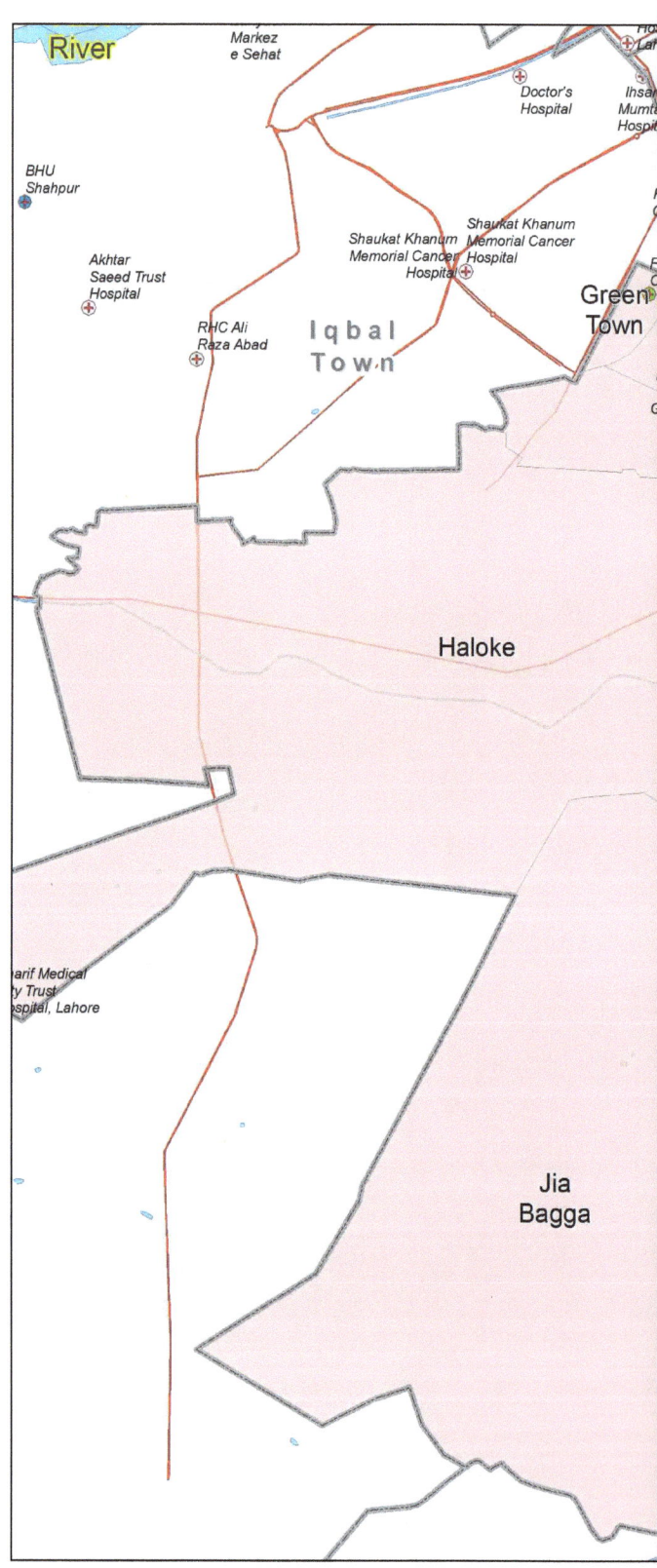

Nishtar Town: Union Council wise summary

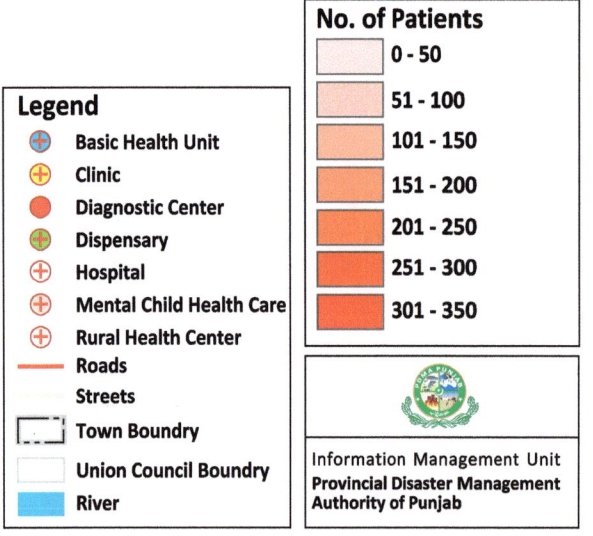

Legend

⊕	Basic Health Unit
⊕	Clinic
●	Diagnostic Center
⊕	Dispensary
⊕	Hospital
⊕	Mental Child Health Care
⊕	Rural Health Center
—	Roads
	Streets
	Town Boundry
	Union Council Boundry
	River

No. of Patients

	0 - 50
	51 - 100
	101 - 150
	151 - 200
	201 - 250
	251 - 300
	301 - 350

Information Management Unit
Provincial Disaster Management Authority of Punjab

Fig: 11

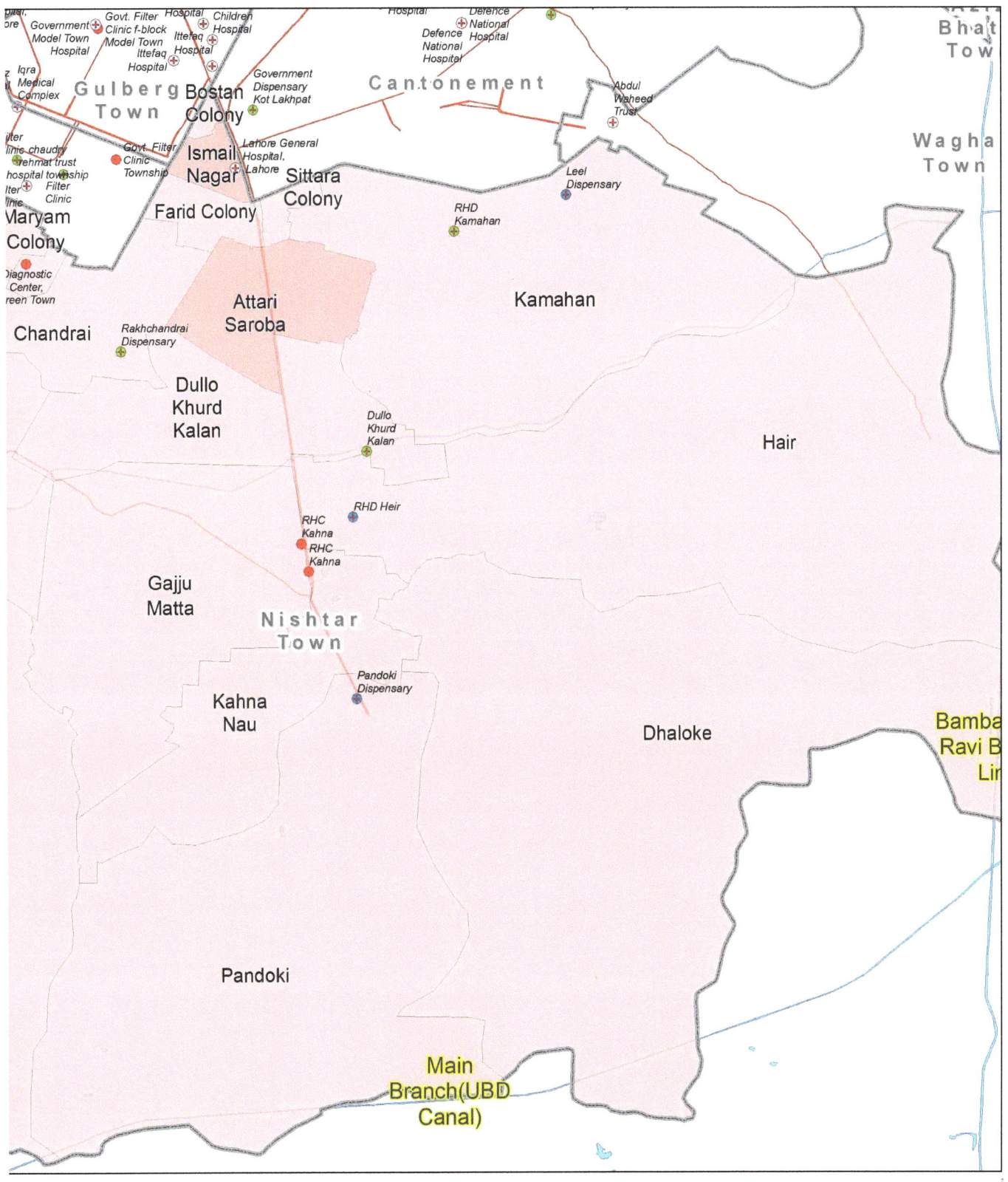

Wagha Town

Compared to other towns of Lahore, Wagha Town was the least affected. Wagha has a large geographic area with a significantly low population density. The only areas that had Dengue patients before the end of September 2011 were Daroghewala and Bhaseen. These areas are along the GT road, and had seen less than 25 cases per Union Council. Despite the low incidence of Dengue fever in this town, the TMA of Wagha Town was proactive in conducting Fogging, Larviciding and IRS across the town.

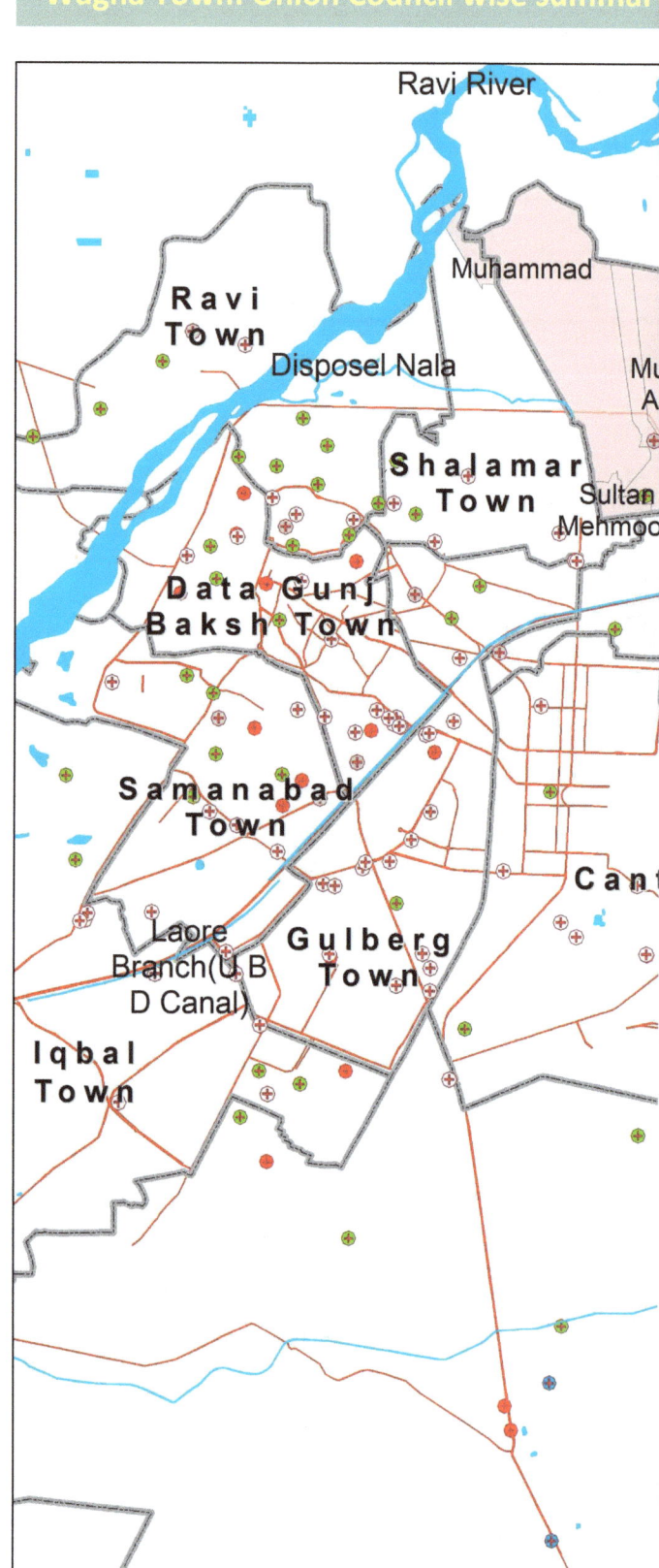

Wagha Town: Union Council wise summary

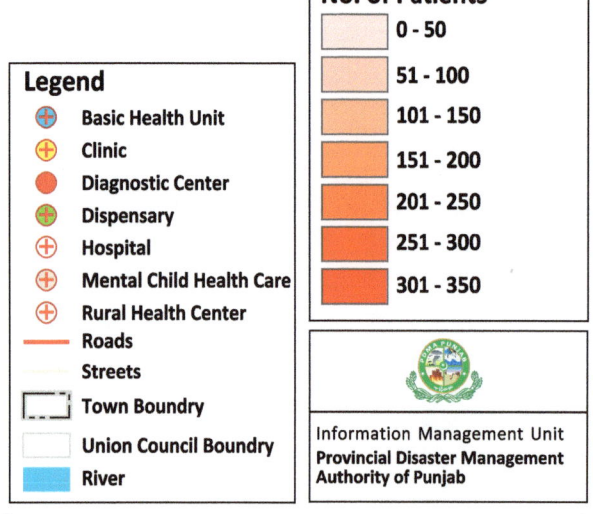

Legend
- 🔵 Basic Health Unit
- 🟡 Clinic
- 🔴 Diagnostic Center
- 🟢 Dispensary
- ⊕ Hospital
- ⊕ Mental Child Health Care
- ⊕ Rural Health Center
- — Roads
- ⋯ Streets
- ▭ Town Boundry
- ▭ Union Council Boundry
- 🟦 River

No. of Patients
- 0 - 50
- 51 - 100
- 101 - 150
- 151 - 200
- 201 - 250
- 251 - 300
- 301 - 350

Information Management Unit
Provincial Disaster Management Authority of Punjab

of Dengue fever cases as of Sept. 30, 2011 *Fig: 12*

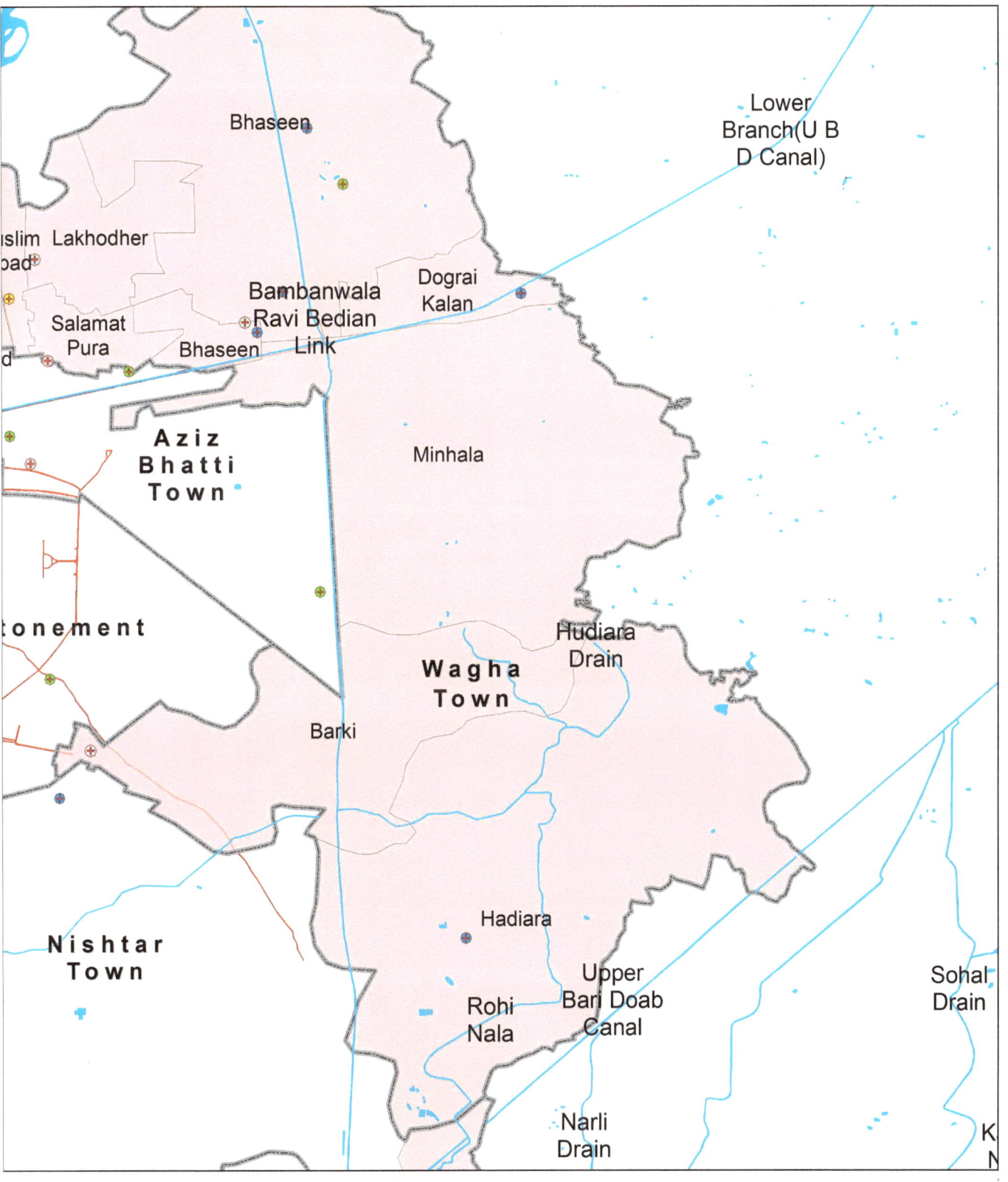

Shalimar Town

Shalimar Town was also one of the less affected towns of Lahore. The Union Council that showed the highest number of patients was Bhagat Pura with 25 positive cases before the end of September 2011. Bhagat Pura is adjacent to Shadbagh which had around 15 cases of this fever.

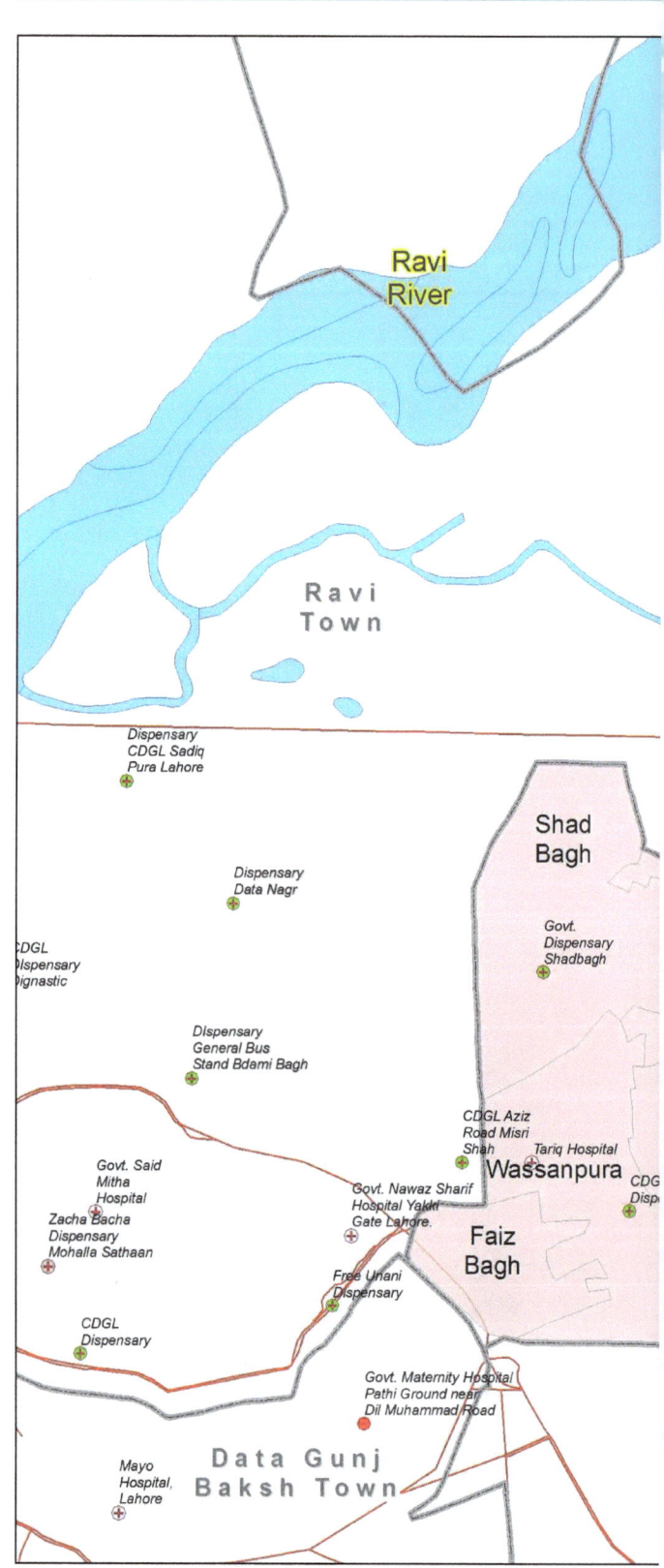

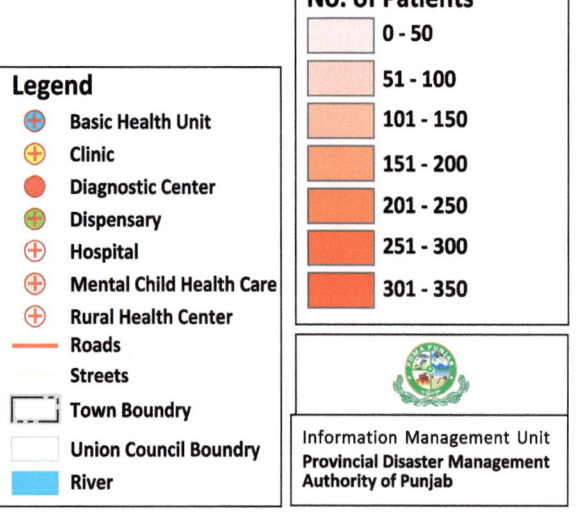

No. of Patients	
	0 - 50
	51 - 100
	101 - 150
	151 - 200
	201 - 250
	251 - 300
	301 - 350

Legend

⊕	Basic Health Unit
⊕	Clinic
●	Diagnostic Center
⊕	Dispensary
⊕	Hospital
⊕	Mental Child Health Care
⊕	Rural Health Center
—	Roads
	Streets
⌐_⌐	Town Boundry
	Union Council Boundry
	River

Information Management Unit
Provincial Disaster Management Authority of Punjab

ary of Dengue fever cases as of Sept. 30, 2011   *Fig: 13*

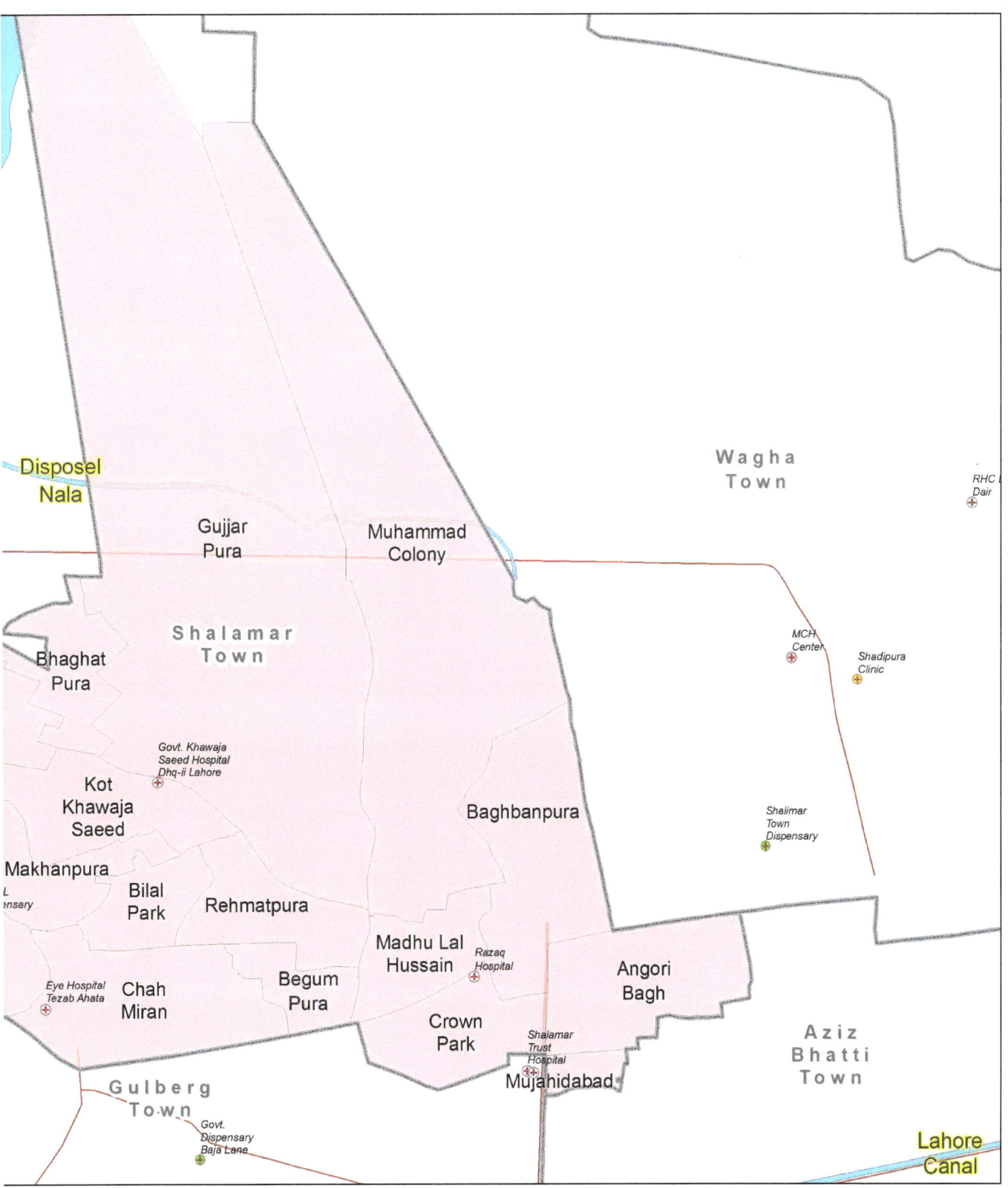

Ravi Town

Ravi Town constitutes the old Lahore. Some of the establishments in this town date back to centuries. The walled city of Lahore, Shahdara and the Fruit Mandi, all lie within this town. Due to the gradual wear and tear, it is not hard to find examples of dilapidated infrastructure. The pollution levels are also high in this town. The open drainage system in certain areas of the old city creates an unhealthy environment. However, the poor drainage system or the high level of pollution did not contribute to the spreading of Dengue virus in this town.

Aedes mosquitoes do not thrive in dirty or polluted humid areas and therefore the incidence of this fever was not as high in this particular town. The walled city of Lahore has the highest population density in the city. The outbreak of a communicable disease in this densely packed community can have a devastating impact. However the spread of Dengue was not as rapid in this area. This can be attributed to the low population levels of *Aedes* mosquitoes in this town. The worst affected Union Council of this town was Rang Mahal. More than sixty residents of this Union Council had been affected with Dengue fever by the end of September 2011.

Legend

- Basic Health Unit
- Clinic
- Diagnostic Center
- Dispensary
- Hospital
- Mental Child Health Care
- Rural Health Center
- Roads
- Streets
- Town Boundry
- Union Council Boundry
- River

No. of Patients

- 0 - 50
- 51 - 100
- 101 - 150
- 151 - 200
- 201 - 250
- 251 - 300
- 301 - 350

Information Management Unit
Provincial Disaster Management Authority of Punjab

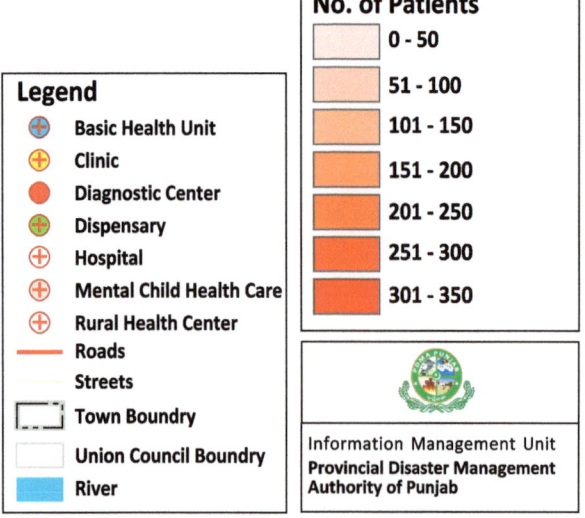

f Dengue fever cases as of Sept. 30, 2011

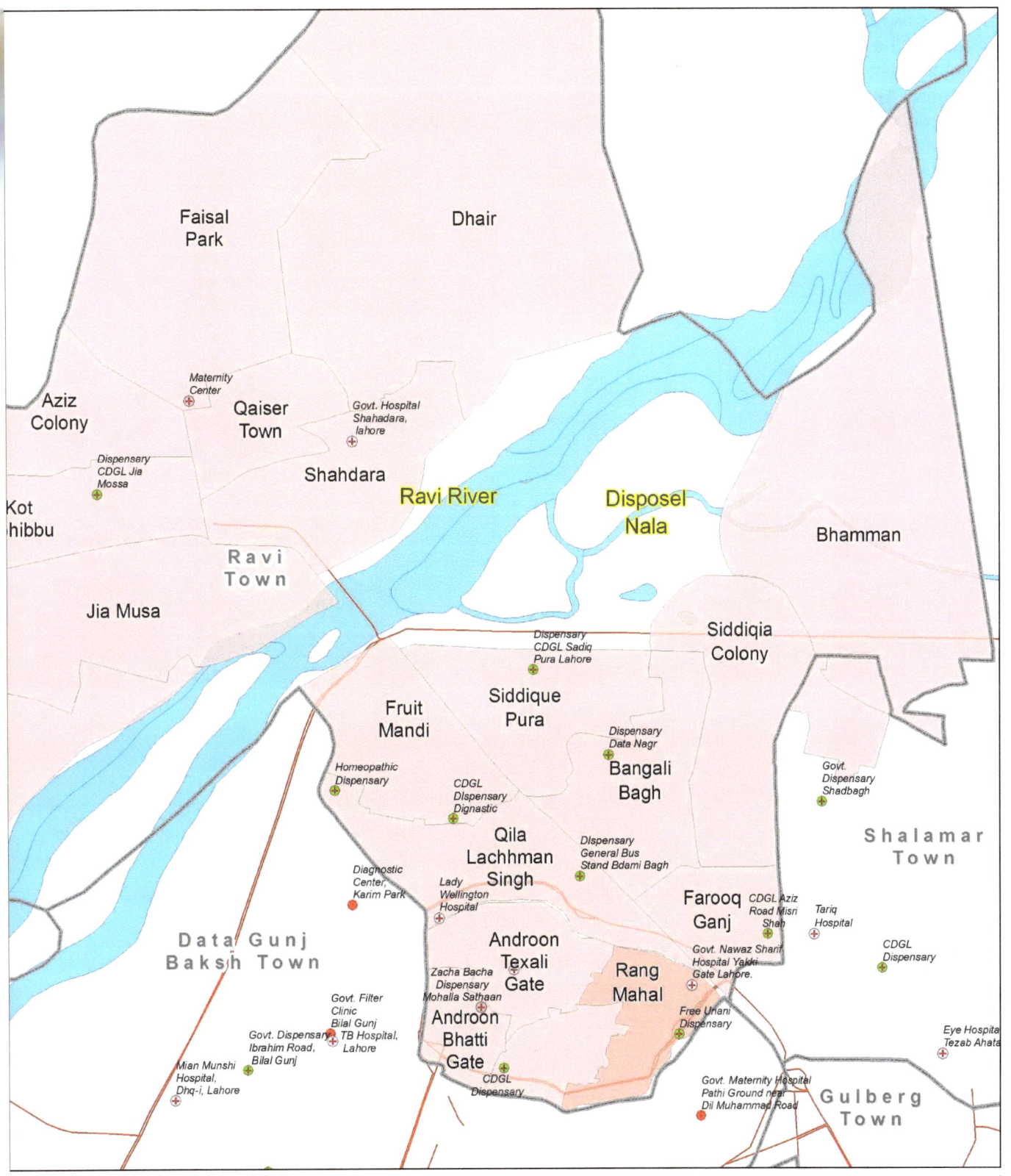

Faisal
Park

Dhair

Maternity
Center

Aziz
Colony

Qaiser
Town

Govt. Hospital
Shahadara,
lahore

Dispensary
CDGL Jia
Mossa

Shahdara

Ravi River

Disposel
Nala

Kot
hibbu

Bhamman

R a v i
T o w n

Jia Musa

Siddiqia
Colony

Dispensary
CDGL Sadiq
Pura Lahore

Fruit
Mandi

Siddique
Pura

Dispensary
Data Nagr

Homeopathic
Dispensary

CDGL
DIspensary
Dignastic

Bangali
Bagh

Govt.
Dispensary
Shadbagh

Qila
Lachhman
Singh

DIspensary
General Bus
Stand Bdami Bagh

S h a l a m a r
T o w n

Diagnostic
Center,
Karim Park

Lady
Wellington
Hospital

Farooq
Ganj

CDGL Aziz
Road Misri
Shah

Tariq
Hospital

D a t a   G u n j
B a k s h   T o w n

Androon
Texali
Gate

Govt. Nawaz Sharif
Hospital Yakki
Gate Lahore.

CDGL
Dispensary

Zacha Bacha
Dispensary
Mohalla Sathaan

Rang
Mahal

Govt. Filter
Clinic
Bilal Gunj

Androon
Bhatti
Gate

Free Unani
Dispensary

Eye Hospita
Tezab Ahata

Govt. Dispensary
Ibrahim Road,
Bilal Gunj

TB Hospital,
Lahore

Mian Munshi
Hospital,
Dhq-i, Lahore

CDGL
Dispensary

Govt. Maternity Hospital
Pathi Ground near
Dil Muhammad Road

G u l b e r g
T o w n

Allama Iqbal Town

Allama Iqbal Town is a geographically large town suggesting a low population density. The two major population centers in this town are Johar Town and Township. Both of these areas had generated more than hundred patients of Dengue fever before the end of September 2011. Dengue patients in the Manga Union Council, which is also an Urban Area, were negligible.

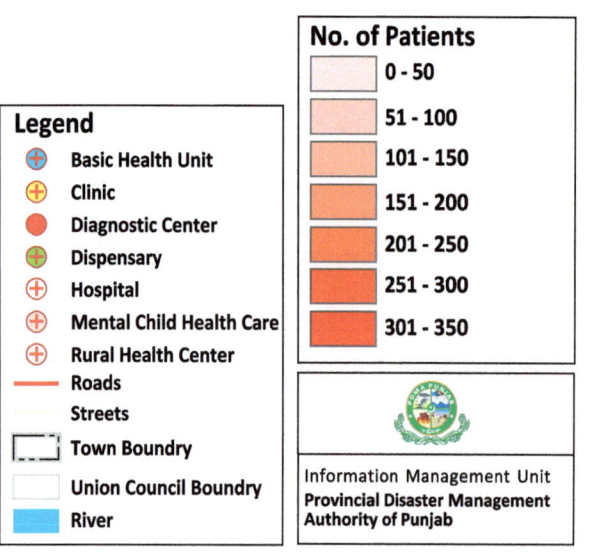

Legend
- ⊕ Basic Health Unit
- ⊕ Clinic
- 🔴 Diagnostic Center
- ⊕ Dispensary
- ⊕ Hospital
- ⊕ Mental Child Health Care
- ⊕ Rural Health Center
- — Roads
- Streets
- ☐ Town Boundry
- ☐ Union Council Boundry
- ▇ River

No. of Patients
- 0 - 50
- 51 - 100
- 101 - 150
- 151 - 200
- 201 - 250
- 251 - 300
- 301 - 350

Information Management Unit
Provincial Disaster Management Authority of Punjab

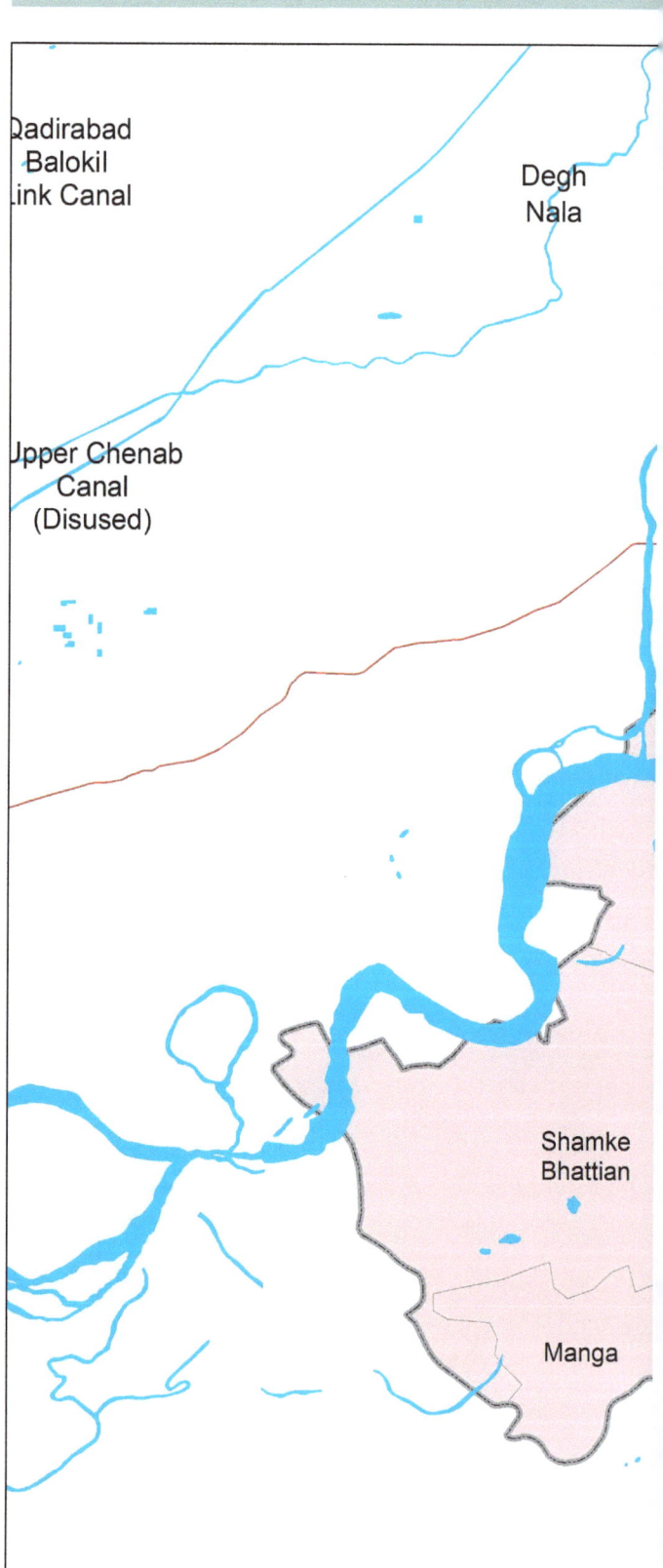

Allama Iqbal Town: Union Council wise sun

Qadirabad Balokil Link Canal

Degh Nala

Upper Chenab Canal (Disused)

Shamke Bhattian

Manga

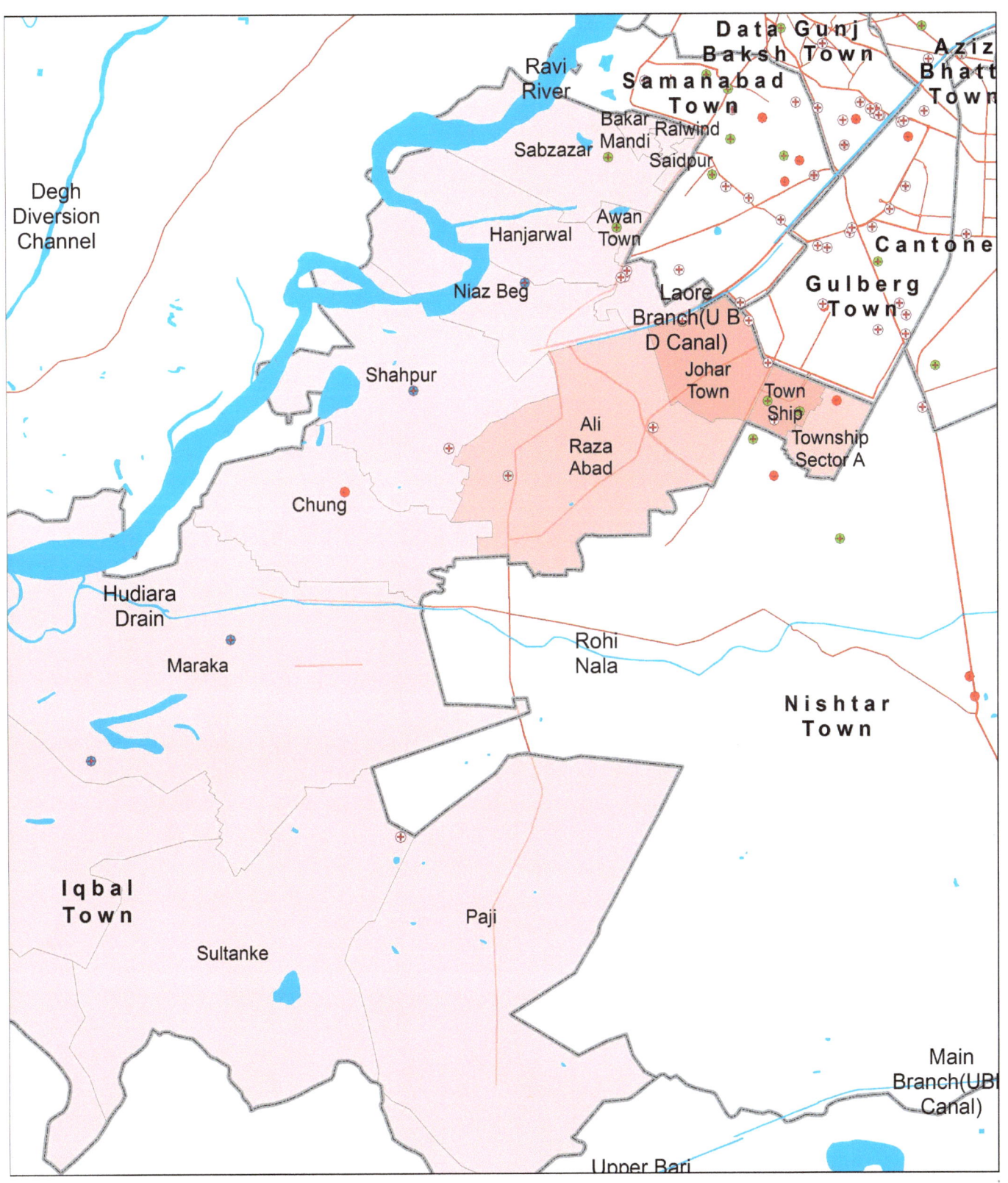

Samnabad Town

Samnabad Town had a relatively high incidence of Dengue fever. More than 167 patients were diagnosed with this fever in the Ichra area alone. The Union Council of Ichra borders the Race Course Union Council of Data Gunj Buksh Town. Race Course had about 200 patients of Dengue fever before the end of September 2011. Apart from Ichra, areas such as Muslim Town, Samnabad and Gulshan-e-Ravi were also affected.

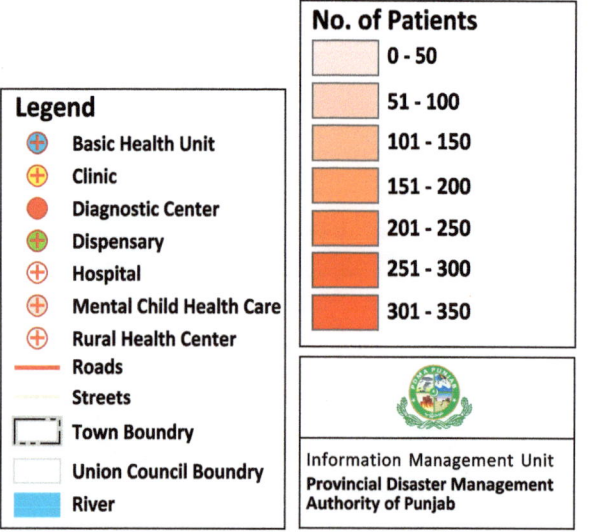

No. of Patients

	0 - 50
	51 - 100
	101 - 150
	151 - 200
	201 - 250
	251 - 300
	301 - 350

Legend

- ⊕ Basic Health Unit
- ⊕ Clinic
- ● Diagnostic Center
- ⊕ Dispensary
- ⊕ Hospital
- ⊕ Mental Child Health Care
- ⊕ Rural Health Center
- — Roads
- Streets
- [ ] Town Boundry
- [ ] Union Council Boundry
- ▬ River

Information Management Unit
Provincial Disaster Management Authority of Punjab

nary of Dengue fever cases as of Sept. 30, 2011 *Fig: 16*

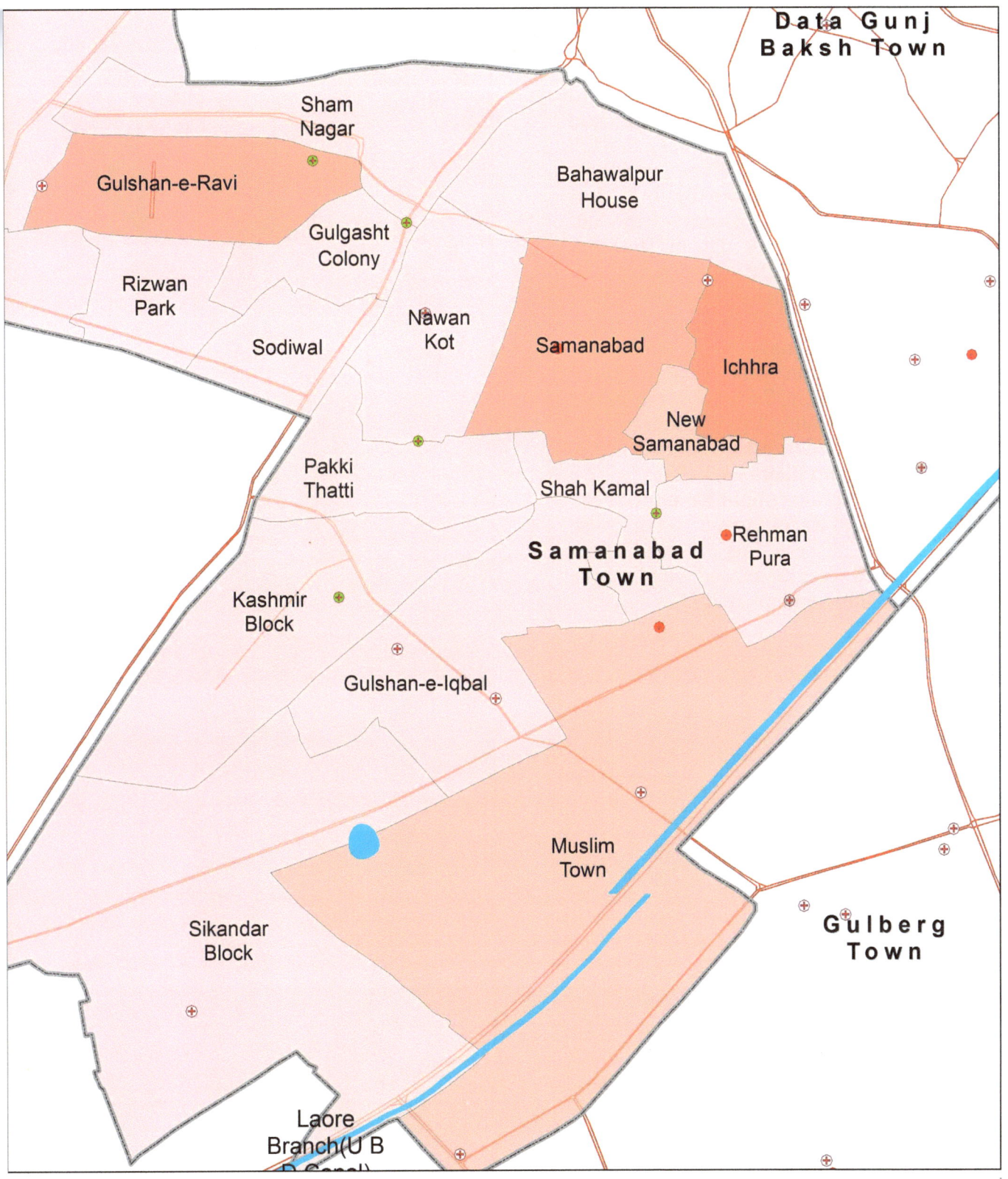

Data Gunj Buksh Town

Data Gunj Buksh Town was one of the worst affected towns of Lahore. More than 200 cases of Dengue fever were reported from the Mozang area of this town. Mozang is home to Miani Sahib, the largest graveyard of Lahore. Grave-diggers in Miani Sahib had built multiple water ponds across the 150 acre graveyard. Water from these ponds was used to soften the soil before digging. Most of the water ponds in this graveyard had larvae of *Aedes* mosquitoes in them. The Local Government Department conducted a comprehensive fumigation of this graveyard at the end of September 2011. Their timely action apparently checked the further spread of this disease in Mozang and other adjacent Union Councils of Data Gunj Buksh Town. Mozang borders the Race Course Union Council which contains the two largest parks of Lahore: Jinnah Garden and Jillani Park (Race Course Park). Monsoon rains might have produced ideal habitats of *Aedes* Mosquitoes in these parks. About 200 residents of Race Course Union Council were diagnosed with Dengue fever before 30th September 2011.

Data Gunj Buksh Town: Union Council wise

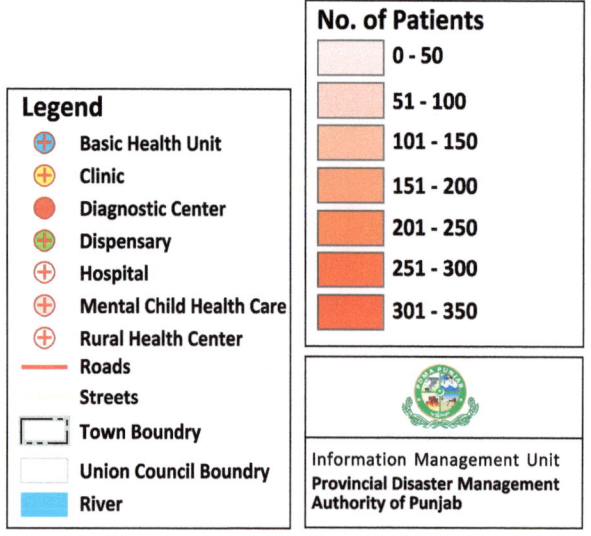

Ravi Town

Kareer Park

Dat Baks

Chohan Park

Ravi River

Sanda Kalan

Jamiyyat Trust Hospital

Legend

- ⊕ Basic Health Unit
- ⊕ Clinic
- ● Diagnostic Center
- ⊕ Dispensary
- ⊕ Hospital
- ⊕ Mental Child Health Care
- ⊕ Rural Health Center
- — Roads
- Streets
- Town Boundry
- Union Council Boundry
- River

No. of Patients

- 0 - 50
- 51 - 100
- 101 - 150
- 151 - 200
- 201 - 250
- 251 - 300
- 301 - 350

Information Management Unit
Provincial Disaster Management Authority of Punjab

summary of Dengue fever cases as of Sept. 30, 2011

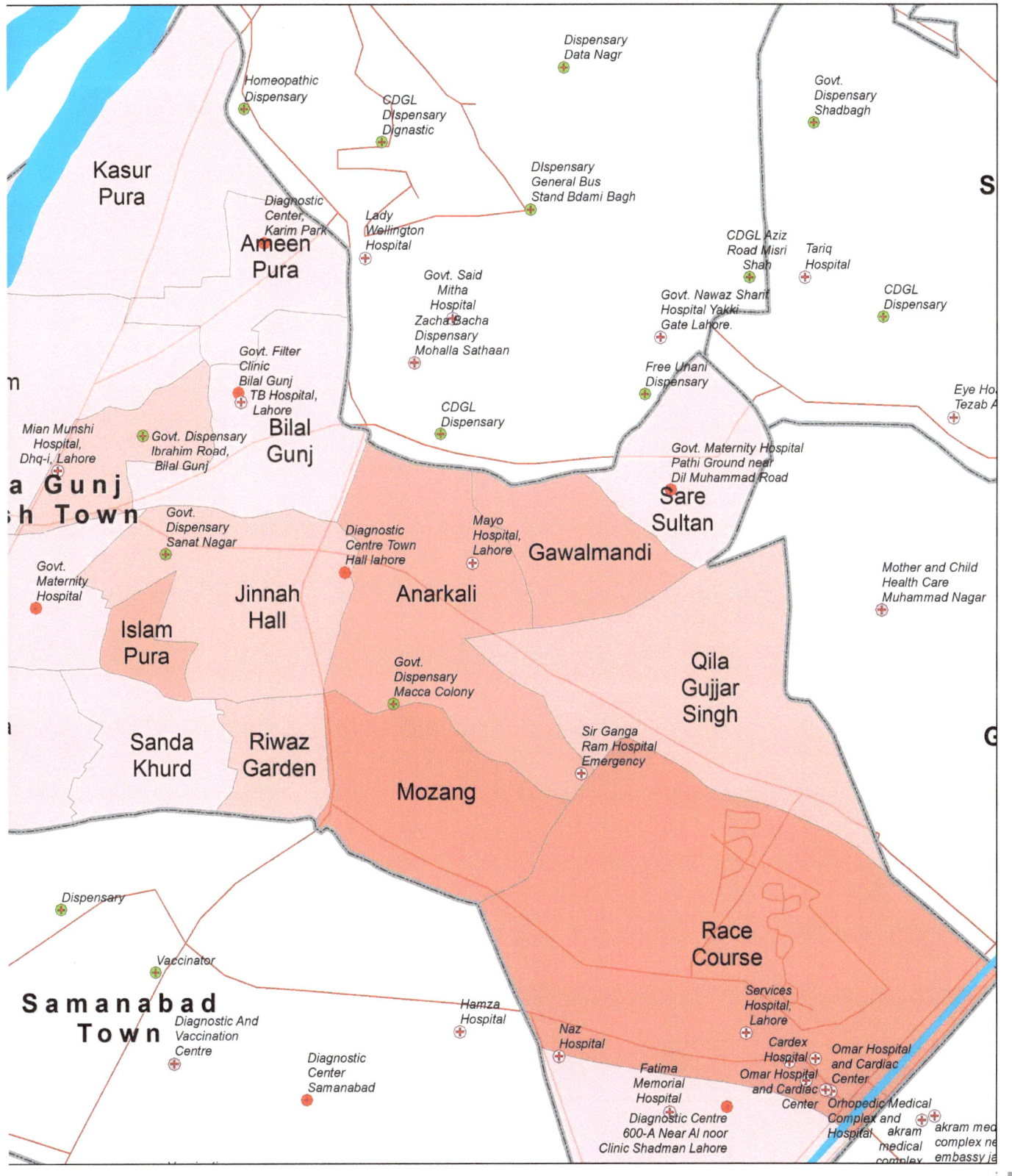

Gulberg Town

Gulberg Town had a high incidence of Dengue fever. However the spread of this disease was fairly irregular. Most of the Union Councils in this town had less than 60 patients of Dengue fever with Faisal Town and Garden Town going up to 100 cases in their respective Union Councils. The single outlier, however, was Model Town which had more than 300 Dengue fever cases before 30th September 2011. Ideal vector habitats in Model Town Park might have resulted in such a high number of patients. Model Town is the worst affected Union Council of the entire city (after excluding Cantonment).

Cantonment

The Cantonment Area has a different administrative setup and the area under its jurisdiction is not divided into Union Councils. As a result a similar analysis of this area was not possible. The data on patients from this area revealed that a large proportion of patients resided in the Defence Housing Authority. About 1,200 cases of Dengue fever were reported from Cantonment before the end of September 2011. Other than Cantonment, it was only Data Gunj Buksh Town which reported a similarly high number of patients.

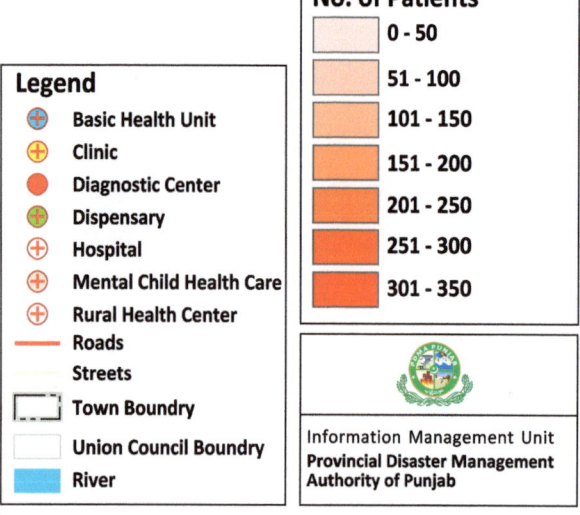

Legend

⊕	Basic Health Unit
⊕	Clinic
●	Diagnostic Center
⊕	Dispensary
⊕	Hospital
⊕	Mental Child Health Care
⊕	Rural Health Center
—	Roads
	Streets
⊏⊐	Town Boundary
☐	Union Council Boundry
▬	River

No. of Patients

	0 - 50
	51 - 100
	101 - 150
	151 - 200
	201 - 250
	251 - 300
	301 - 350

Information Management Unit
Provincial Disaster Management Authority of Punjab

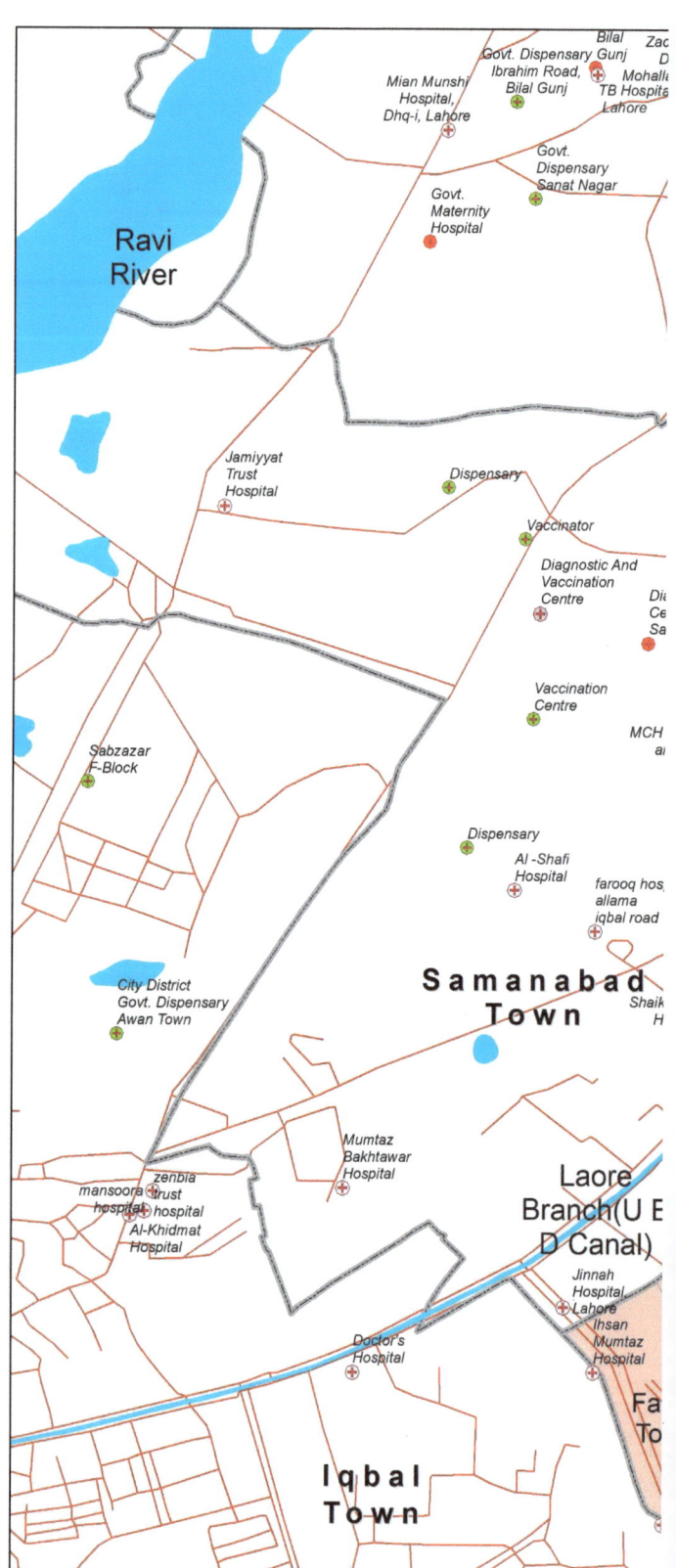

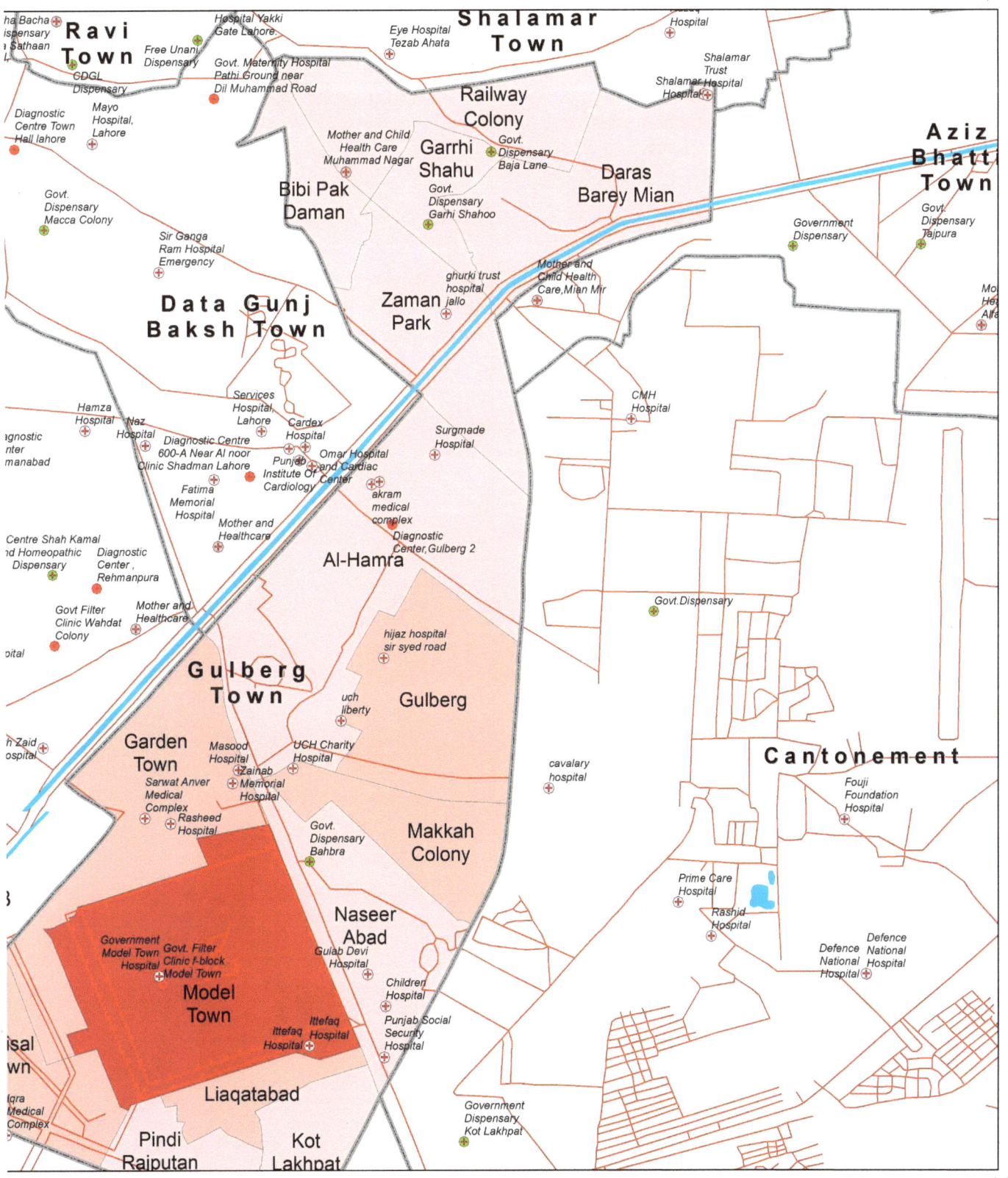

...ry of Dengue fever cases as of Sept. 30, 2011   *Fig: 18*

Comprehensive Map of Lahore

The comprehensive map of Lahore reveals that besides Cantonment the worst affected areas of the city are Model Town, Race Course, Mozang and Ichra. All of the worst affected Union Councils have either Parks or Graveyards in them and it is these areas where the vector colonies had thrived prior to the chemical control of the city.

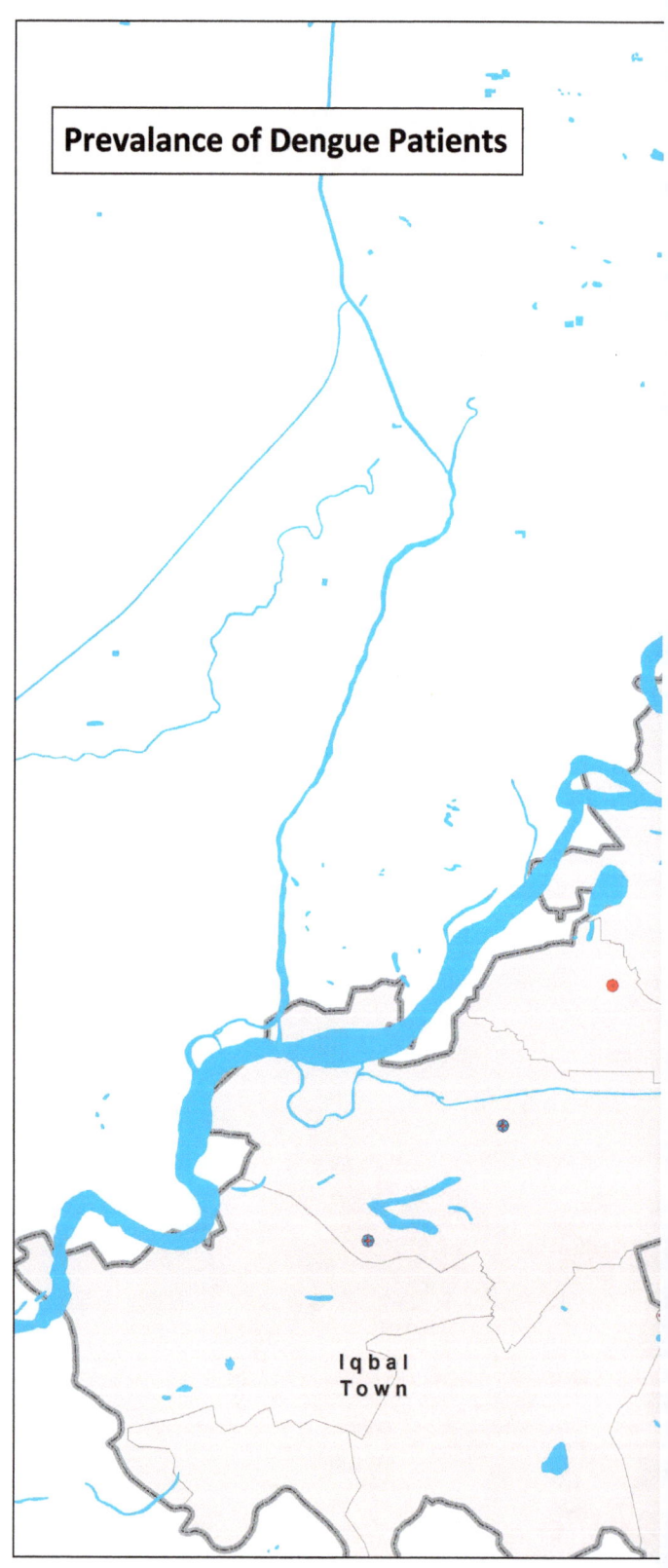

Prevalance of Dengue Patients

Iqbal
Town

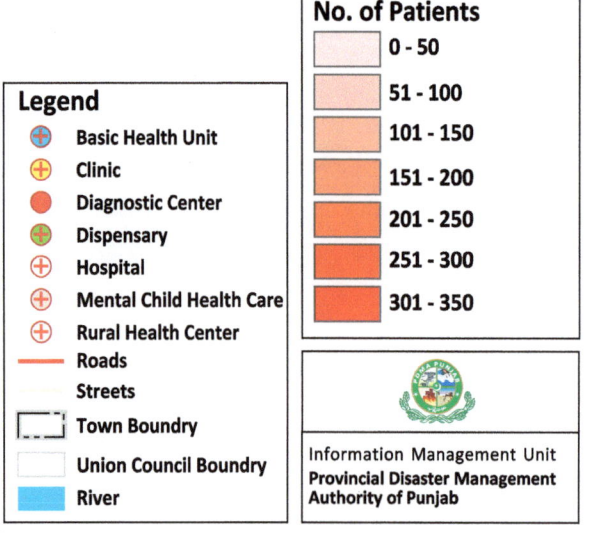

Legend

⊕	Basic Health Unit
⊕	Clinic
●	Diagnostic Center
⊕	Dispensary
⊕	Hospital
⊕	Mental Child Health Care
⊕	Rural Health Center
—	Roads
	Streets
⊏⊐	Town Boundry
	Union Council Boundry
▮	River

No. of Patients

	0 - 50
	51 - 100
	101 - 150
	151 - 200
	201 - 250
	251 - 300
	301 - 350

Information Management Unit
Provincial Disaster Management Authority of Punjab

ory of Dengue fever cases as of Sept. 30, 2011

Fig: 19

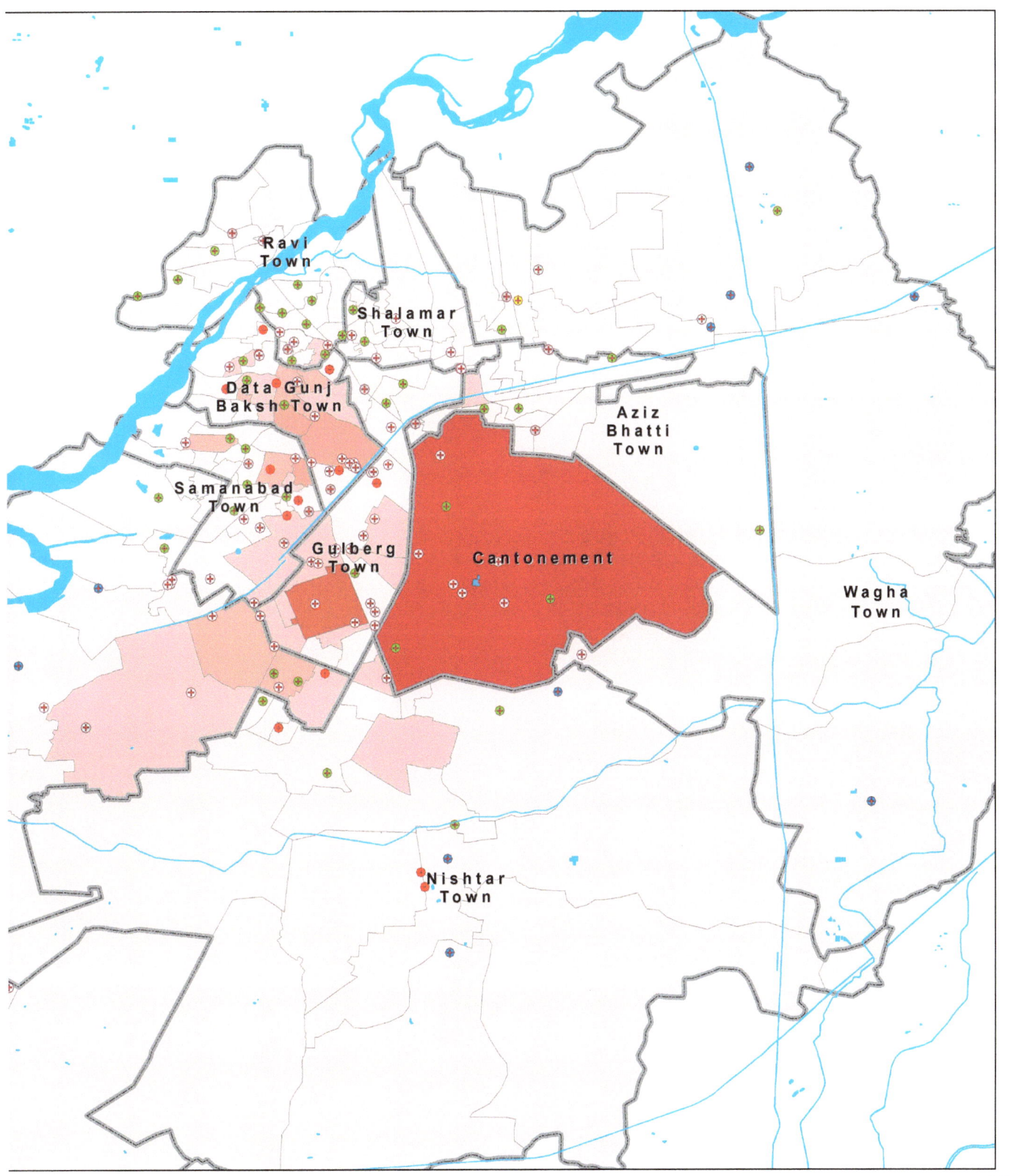

Vector Prevalence

The Agriculture Department mobilized 70 Entomologists to conduct more than 12,000 spot-checks identifying areas that had larvae or adult mosquitoes' presence. These spot-checks were carried out after these areas were fumigated.

PDMA organized the data of these 12,000 spot-checks along with the Union Councils and calculated the percentage of spots for every Union Council where a larva or adult mosquito was found. For example, the Entomologists' team conducted about 100 spot-checks in the Kasur Pura Union Council of Data Gunj Buksh Town. Mosquitoes or larvae were found in only 20 of those 100 spot-checks. PDMA used this data to conclude that the vector prevalence in Kasur Pura Union Council was 20 %.

Figure 20 concludes that the areas which generated highest number of patients before the fumigation was carried out, had significantly lower vector prevalence after the fumigation. Larvae or Adult mosquitoes were found in only 12% of the spot-checks conducted in the Model Town Area. This is considerably low when compared to the Fruit Mandi in Ravi Town where vector was found in 60% of the spot-checks. The low level of vector prevalence in Model Town was an evidence of the fact that the Government of Punjab conducted substantial chemical control in the area, once they were informed of the high number of Dengue patients in Model Town.

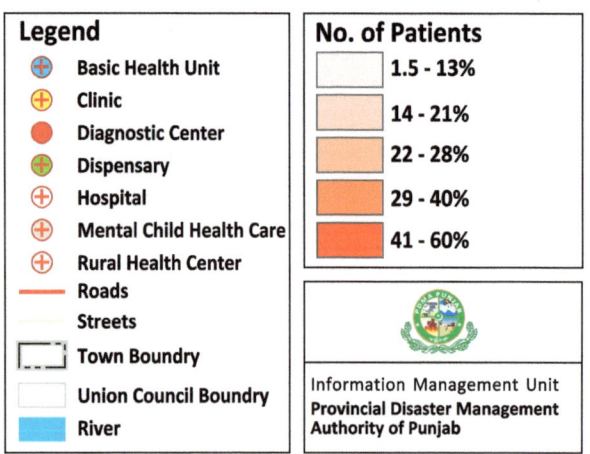

Legend

		No. of Patients	
⊕	Basic Health Unit		1.5 - 13%
⊕	Clinic		14 - 21%
●	Diagnostic Center		22 - 28%
⊕	Dispensary		29 - 40%
⊕	Hospital		41 - 60%
⊕	Mental Child Health Care		
⊕	Rural Health Center		
—	Roads		
	Streets		
	Town Boundary		
	Union Council Boundry		
	River		

Information Management Unit
Provincial Disaster Management Authority of Punjab

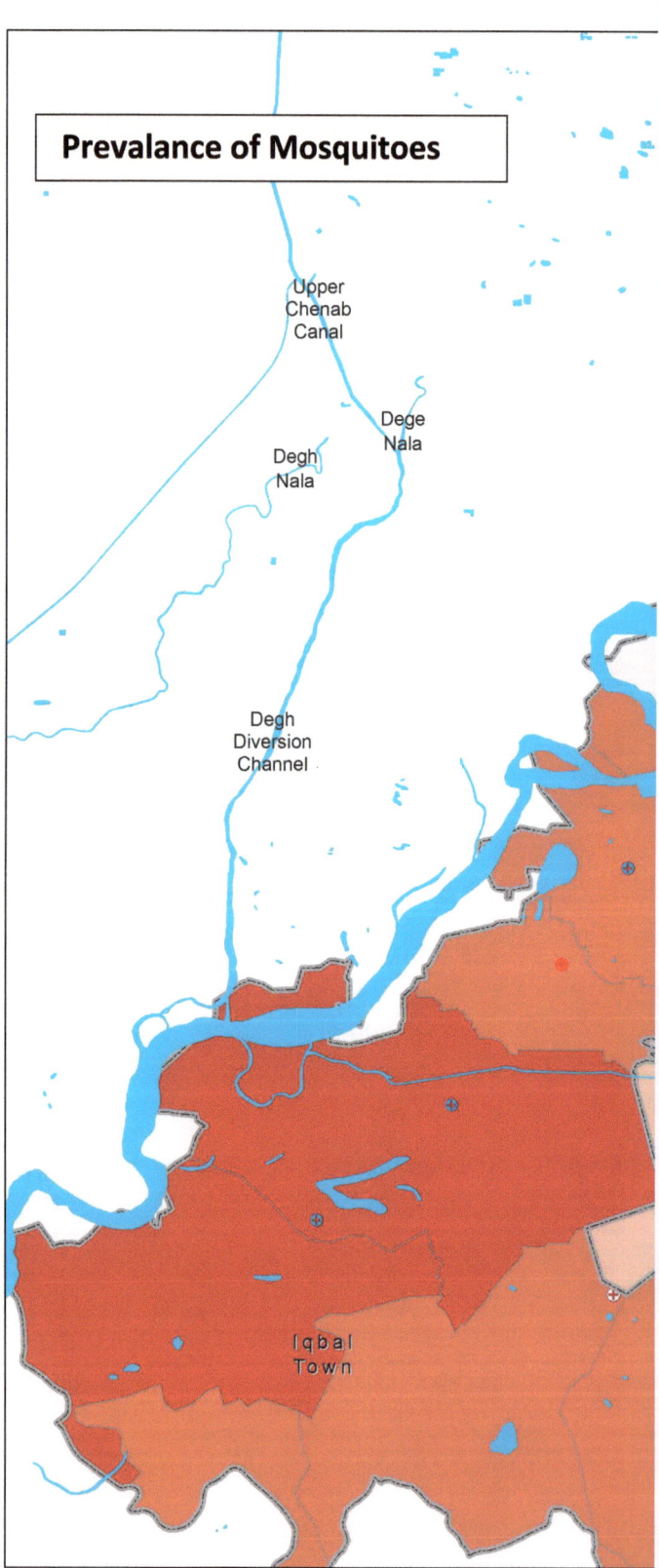

Prevalance of Mosquitoes

Upper Chenab Canal

Dege Nala

Degh Nala

Degh Diversion Channel

Iqbal Town

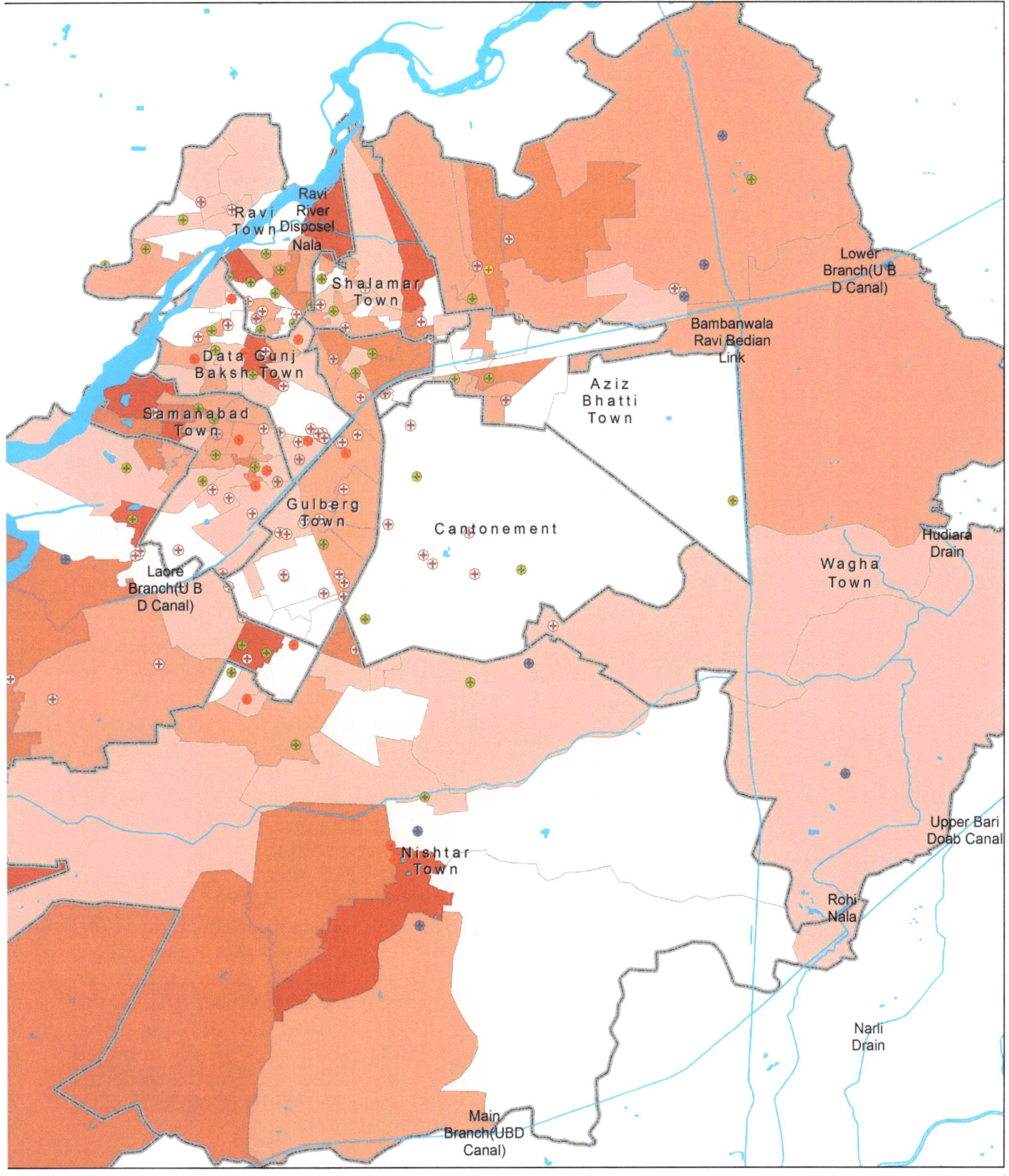

Policy Prescriptions

The following policy prescriptions are derived from the observations made in the research detailed above.

1. The Government of Punjab must initiate an annual fumigation campaign in Parks and Graveyards across Lahore before the onset of each monsoon season or spring

2. Policy guidelines for the prevention and control of Dengue fever should be developed in the light of the prior experiences of the government, as documented in research studies

3. All efforts should be made to eliminate the development of stagnant fresh water ponds and collection of damp or humid debris, as these places act as ideal habitats of *Aedes* mosquitoes

The Correlation between Rainfall and Dengue fever cases

PDMA's GIS analysis concludes that the highest numbers of Dengue cases were observed at areas that had either Parks or Graveyards. Rainfall during the monsoon season created humid breeding spots in the waste foliage or small ponds of Parks and Graveyards. Miani Sahib is a vast Graveyard in the Mozang Union Council. More than 200 patients from this area had been diagnosed with Dengue fever at the peak of the epidemic outbreak. Most of Lahore's other Union Councils had generated less than 50 patients by that time. Mozang saw a disproportionately higher number of Dengue patients due to the presence of mosquito colonies that thrived in the humid environments of the Miani Sahib Graveyard.

The staff of Local Government Department observed the presence of larvae in about 70 water ponds of over hundred acres of this vast Graveyard. The Department later conducted a comprehensive chemical control in this Graveyard.

The Parks and Horticulture Authority fumigated the parks along similar lines. The execution of these fumigations accelerated the controlling of the proliferation of disease.

The Epidemic outbreak of Dengue fever started in the first week of August when about 16 patients were reported in a week's time. Over a period of one and half month this weekly number went up to 3,743. Each day more than 500 patients were diagnosed with this fever in the 38th week of 2011 (Figure 21). In the week following this, the LG&CD Department along with the PHA fumigated the Graveyards and Parks, eliminating the sources of this disease. Unfortunately, the vector populations had spread out to the households by that time. The fumigation in Parks and Graveyards accelerated the decline in number of patients but this decline was gradual as a significant population of *Aedes* Mosquitoes had found favourable breeding spots in people's homes, used tyres and other enclosed humid spots. In a matter of two months the number of Dengue patients came back to controllable figures. The disease escalated in the months of August and September and then declined in the months of October and November 2011.

PDMA concluded that vector populations of *Aedes Aegyptus* and *Aedes Albopictus* are more sensitive to precipitation than they are to temperature. PDMA reached this conclusion after a holistic research conducted utilizing the data provided by Health and Agriculture Departments. The Health Department provided the data on Dengue patients that were diagnosed with that fever between 1st August and 30th September 2011. The data from Agriculture department was compiled by 70 Entomologists after checking 12,000 spots for the presence of Adult mosquitoes or larvae. This data was collected between 21st September and 16th October 2011. Health Department provided the data of approximately 11,000 patients, 5,737 of whom had provided their addresses. This data reflected the escalation of the epidemic outbreak since it was collected at the time when the number of cases was gradually reaching its peak.

The Health Department communicated the addresses to the relevant TMA, which then conducted the Internal Residual Spray (IRS) in the houses of the patients as well as in 28 other homes in the patient's neighborhood. The purpose of the IRS was to contain the further spread of Dengue fever by eliminating any potential vector habitats in the patient's surroundings. Any *Aedes* mosquito in the surrounding of an already infected patient can carry the disease from the patient to any other person bitten by that same mosquito. The Health department was contributing in the containment of the disease as it was collecting the data from various hospitals and medical centers where the patients were diagnosed with Dengue fever.

According to the prescribed SOPs, when the Health department received the data on a patient residing in the Mozang Union Council of the Data Gunj Baksh Town, itwould forward the patient's data to the TMA of Data

Gunj Baksh Town. The TMA then conducted the IRS in 29 adjacent homes in Mozang. The worst affected union councils were being cleaned just as the data on patients was rolling in. After the 38th week of 2011 when the disease had reached its peak, the Agriculture Department sent out teams to check the presence of *Aedes* mosquitoes in various Union Councils of Lahore. Their findings revealed that the worst affected areas such as Mozang did not have any significant populations of mosquitoes anymore. The Government of Punjab had strategically eliminated the source of this disease by conducting chemical control in the Parks, Graveyards and the Houses of the worst affected areas.

The threat of Dengue virus typically decreases as winters set in. The decreasing temperature contributed to the downfall in the number of Dengue cases but it was not the only factor in the control of this epidemic. The defining factor was Government of Punjab's strategic control of Dengue fever through the identification and elimination of vector

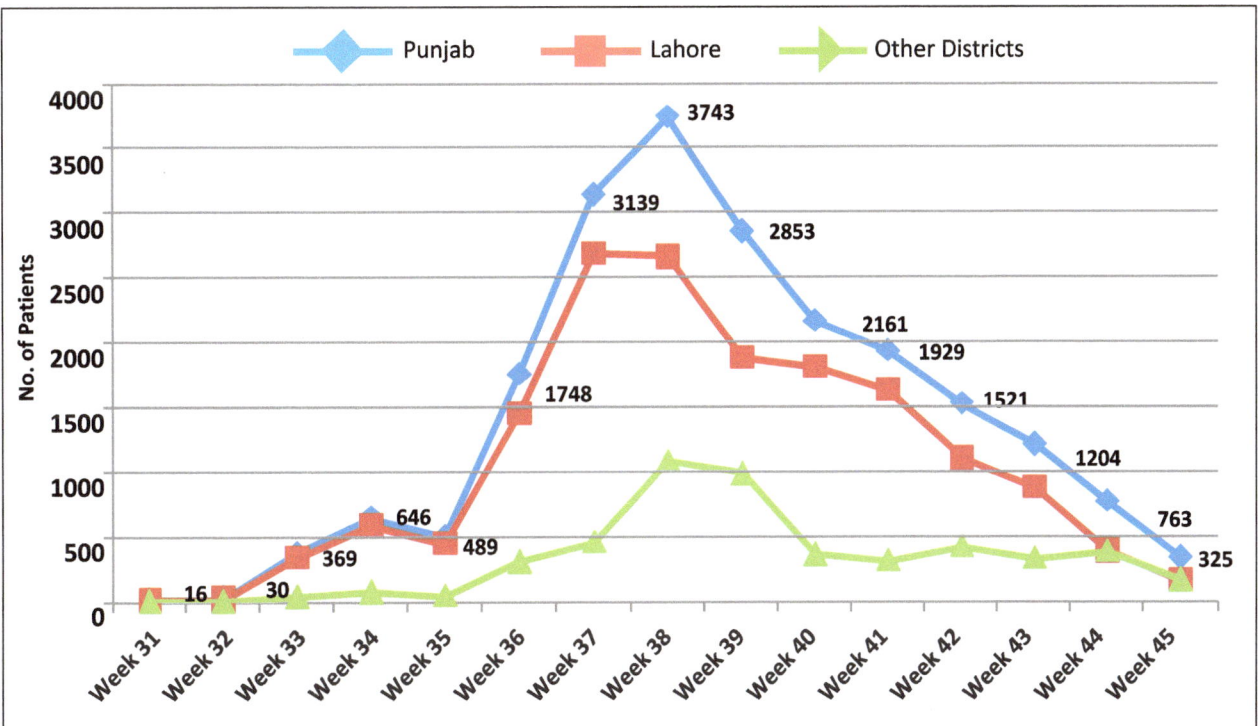

Comparison of Dengue Cases Reported in Lahore and other Districts *Fig. 21*

habitats throughout the city. The Government of Punjab worked to eliminate the source of this disease and such efforts gradually controlled the epidemic outbreak.

The number of Dengue cases started to decrease after the 19th of September 2011. However it was not until the mid of November 2011 that the temperatures became forbiddingly low for *Aedes* Mosquitoes. The Adult mosquitoes of the *Aedei* species become excessively lethargic under 14 °C and even dies if the temperature continues to drop further. The temperature dropped below 14 °C in the mid of November 2011 (Figure 22) and the cold weather eliminated whatever colonies were left despite the massive chemical control. The Government of Punjab had already controlled the source of this disease before the receding temperatures started to assist them in their goal of eliminating the vector population. At the peak of the disease outbreak, Lahore, saw more than 2,600 patients in a week's time. By the mid of November 2011, even before the temperature dropped below

14°C, this number had already fallen to less than 200 patients. Figure 22 shows the minimum temperatures that were recorded in the city of Lahore in the year 2011.

A similar graph for the year 2010 (Figure 23) shows that it was first week of November that the temperature dropped below 14°C. Figure 24 shows the number of weekly cases of Dengue Fever that were recorded in the year 2010. Interestingly, in 2010, the number of cases started to recede after the first week of November 2010, when winter set in, unlike the year 2011 when the decline started much earlier in September.

The Government of Punjab's vector control had checked the epidemic outbreak of the Dengue fever in September, 2011. If the Government had not responded with a massive vector control campaign, the num-ber of patients would have risen till Nov-ember when the receding temperatures eliminate the populations of *Aedes* mosquitoes inhabiting outdoors.

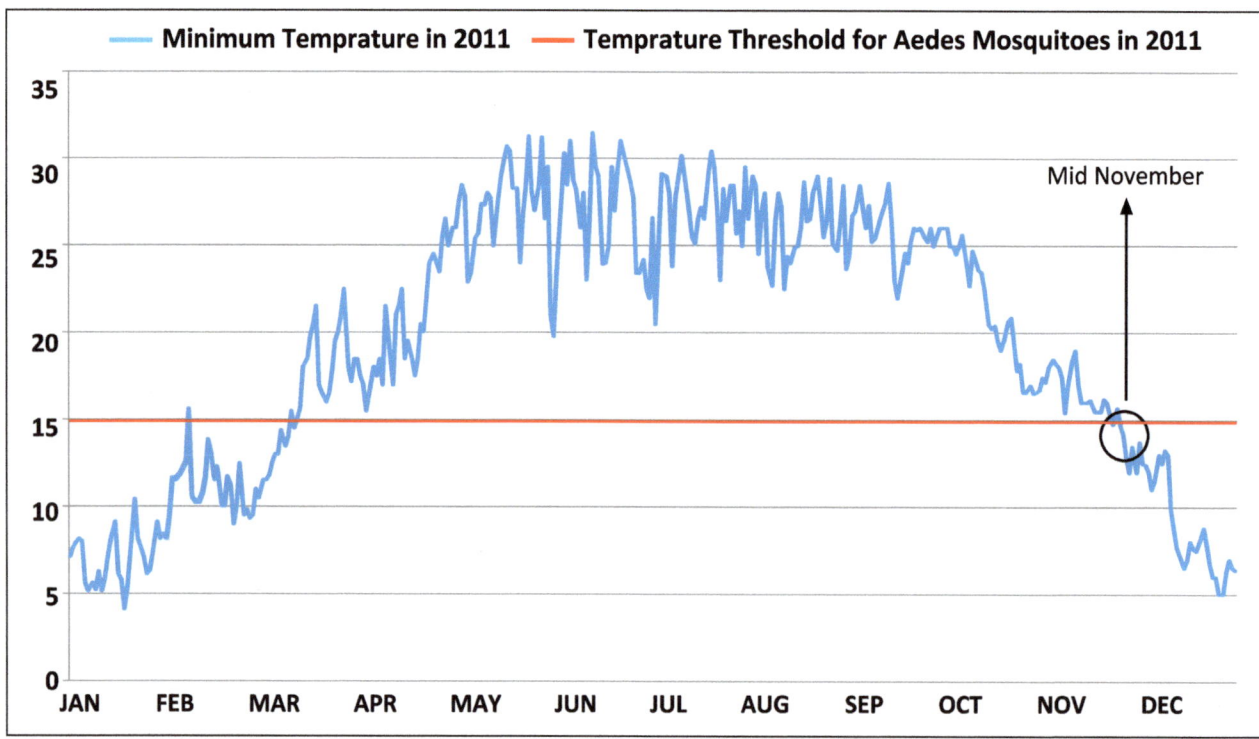

Minimum temperature in 2011   *Fig. 22*

Minimum temperature in 2010
Fig. 23

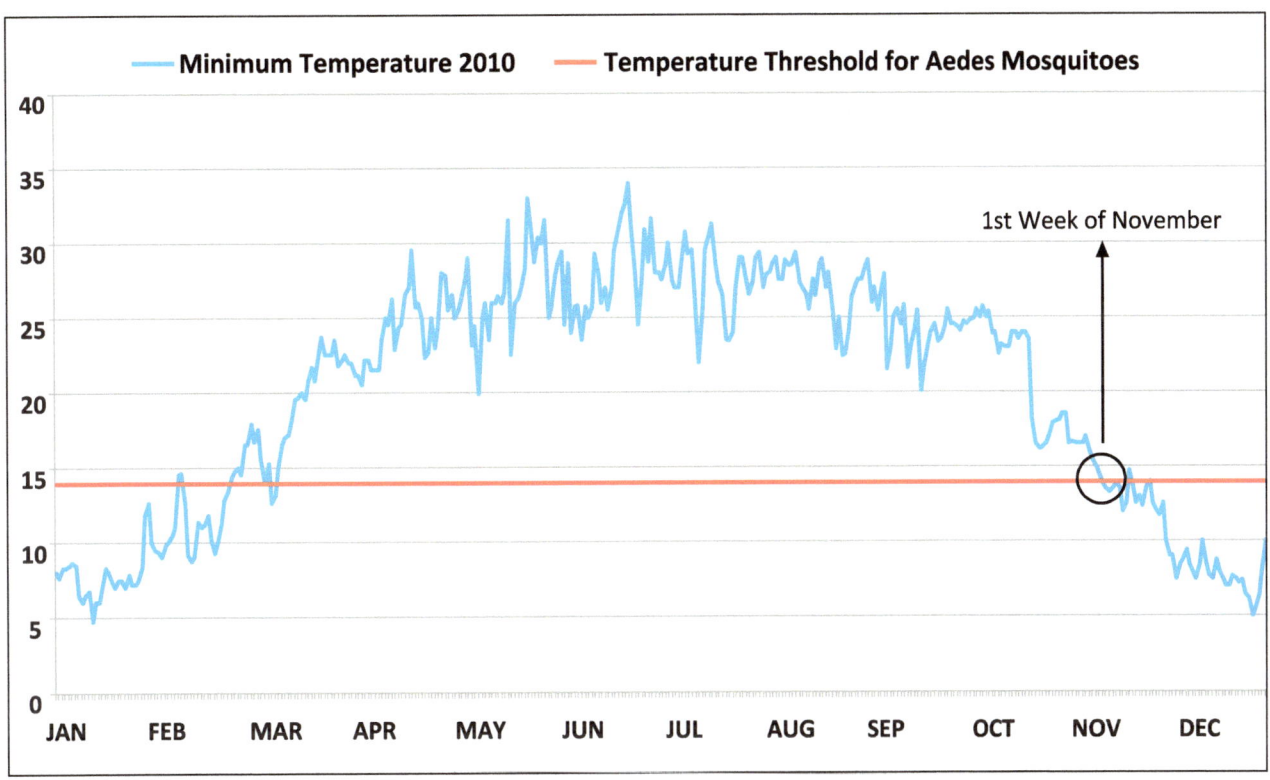

Weekly Dengue Fever Cases recorded in 2010
Fig. 24

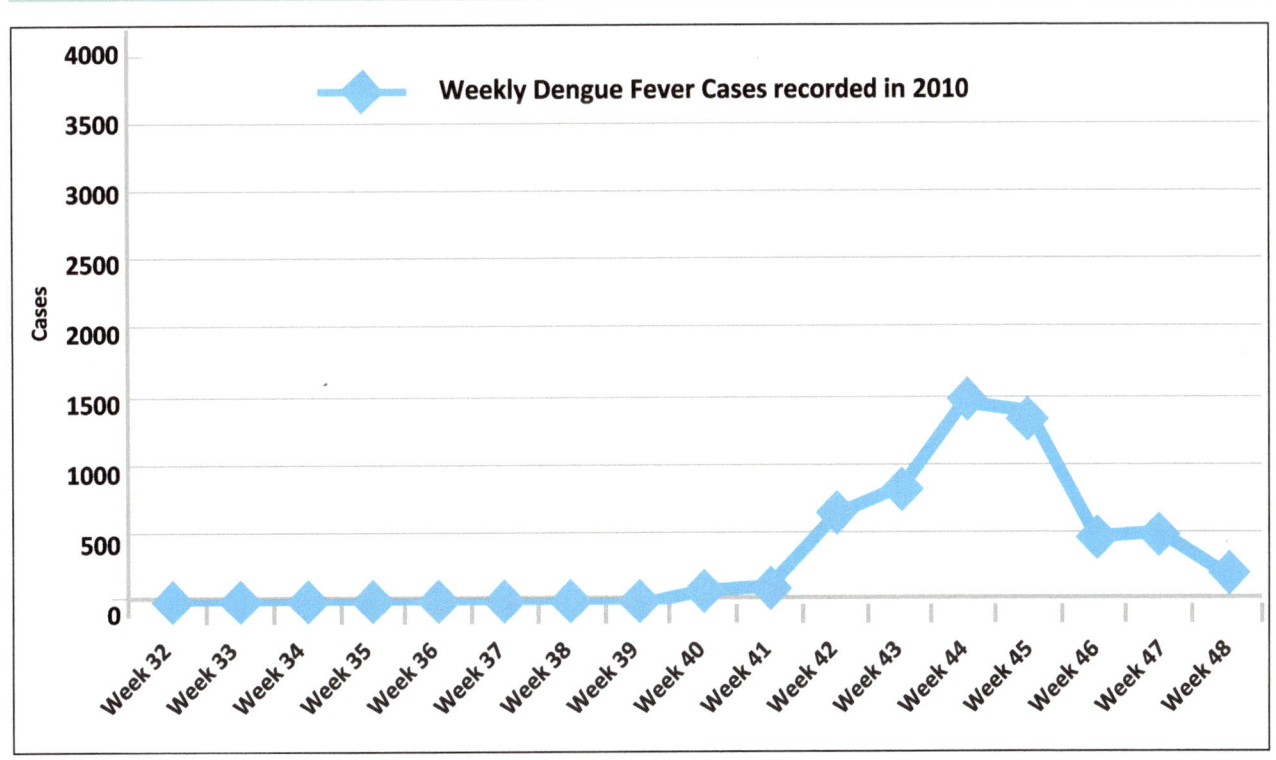

According to Figure 25 the disease would have affected more than 55,000 patients and would have killed about 900 people cumulatively, had the government not checked its proliferation in time. Figure 25 projects the increase in the number of Dengue cases if the governmental intervention was missing. Figure 26 shows that the escalation of this disease was a direct consequence of the rainfall. The city of Lahore saw an urban flooding in the 32nd week of 2011. This flooding due to approximately 13 inches of rainfall created humid spots in the Parks and Graveyards of Lahore.

In a matter of three weeks, the mosquitoes utilized the newly created humid spots to breed in large numbers. The growth in the vector population led to an exponential increase in the number of patients diagnosed with the Dengue fever.

As per this analysis it was only the Government of the Punjab's relentless efforts, which ushered in the decline of the disease through a strategic campaign. After the 38th week when the disease had reached its peak, the government's chemical control in the urban areas of Lahore accelerated the decline in Dengue cases, and government's perseverance in eliminating the hot-spots led to an almost complete elimination of Dengue.

Dengue is a recurring problem in Pakistan. It also affected a significant population in 2010 but that year too the rise in the number of cases was observed after the monsoon rains had created humid spots for mosquitoes to breed.

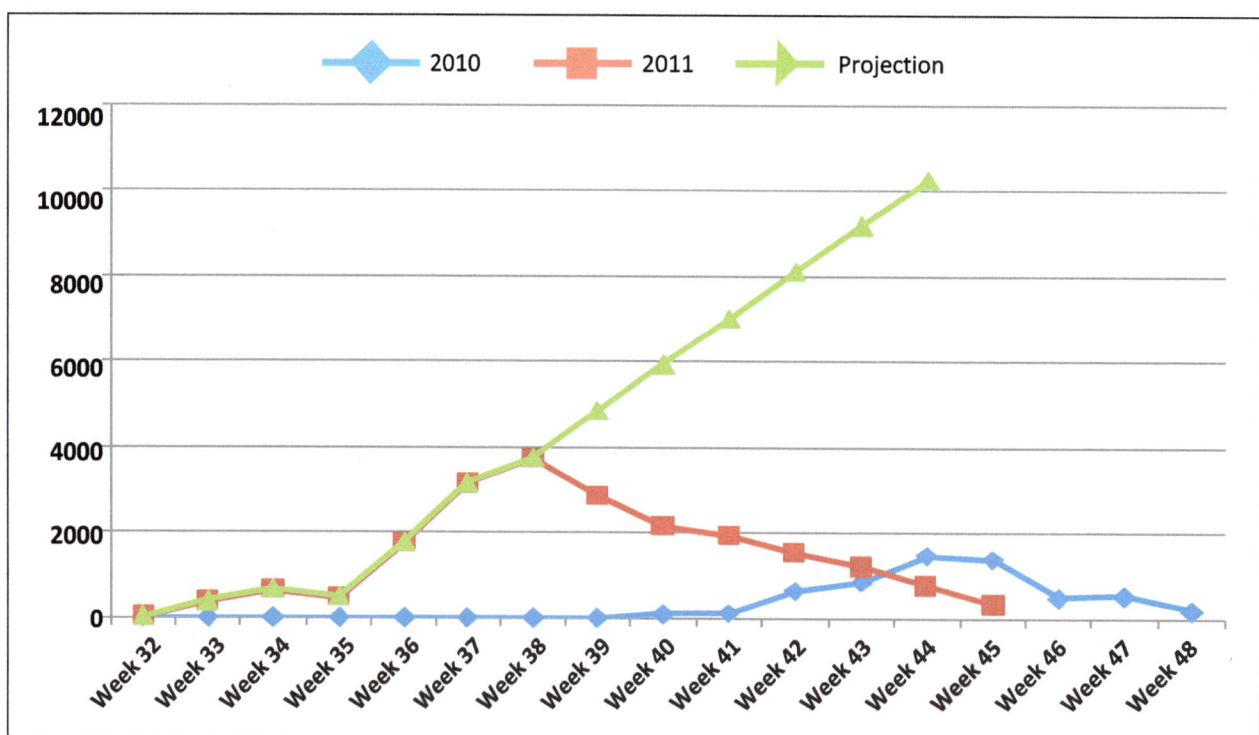

Projection of fever cases   *Fig. 25*

Weekly Dengue Fever Cases recorded in 2011

Fig. 26

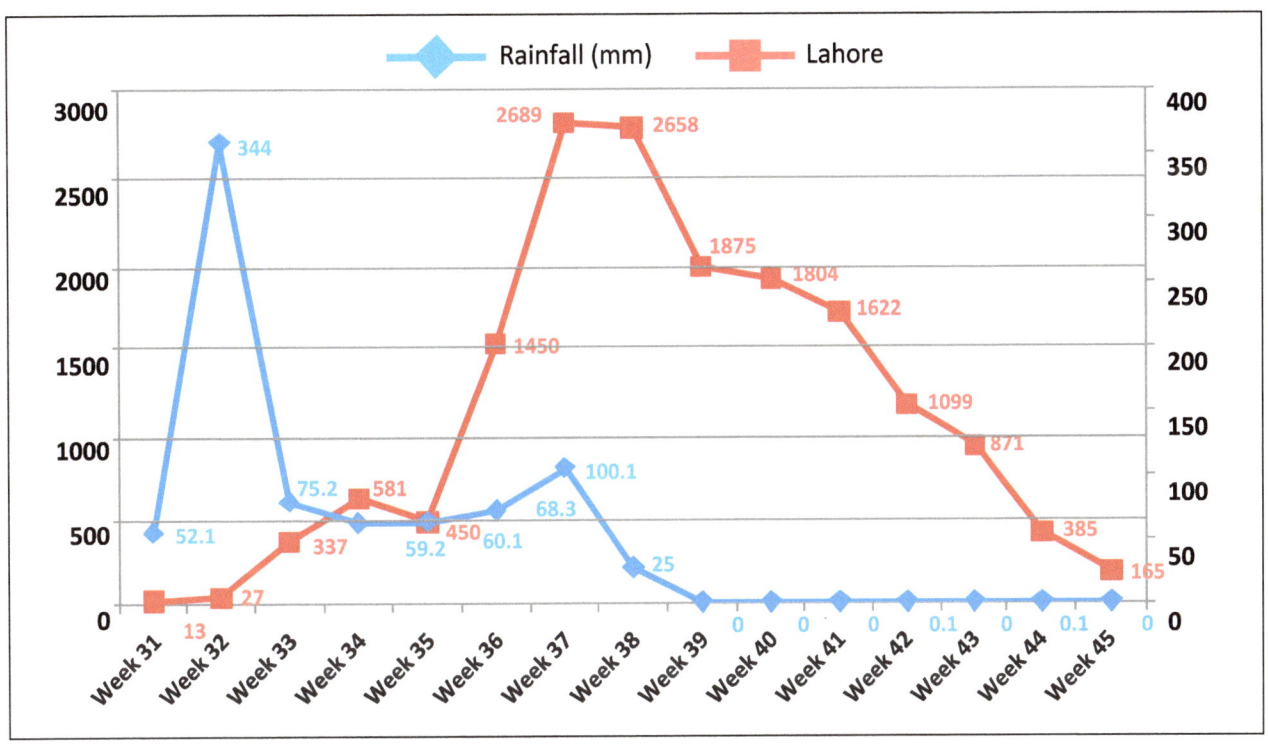

Weekly Comparison of Dengue Cases 2010 - 2011

Fig. 27

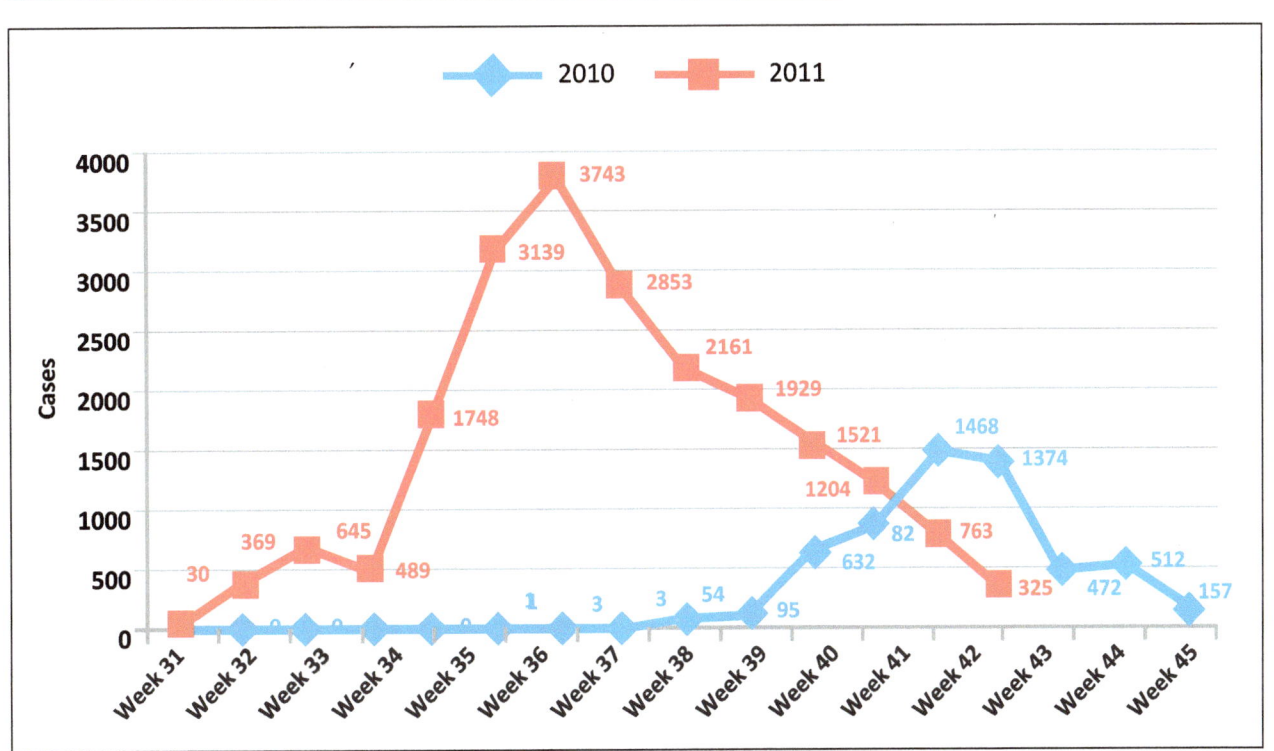

The menace of Dengue also spread to other Districts by the end of 2011 as reflected in Figure 28. The communication of this virus is usually attributed to the high number of people commuting between other cities and Lahore. The monsoon rains also created ideal vector habitats in other cities, contributing to the province wide proliferation of this disease.

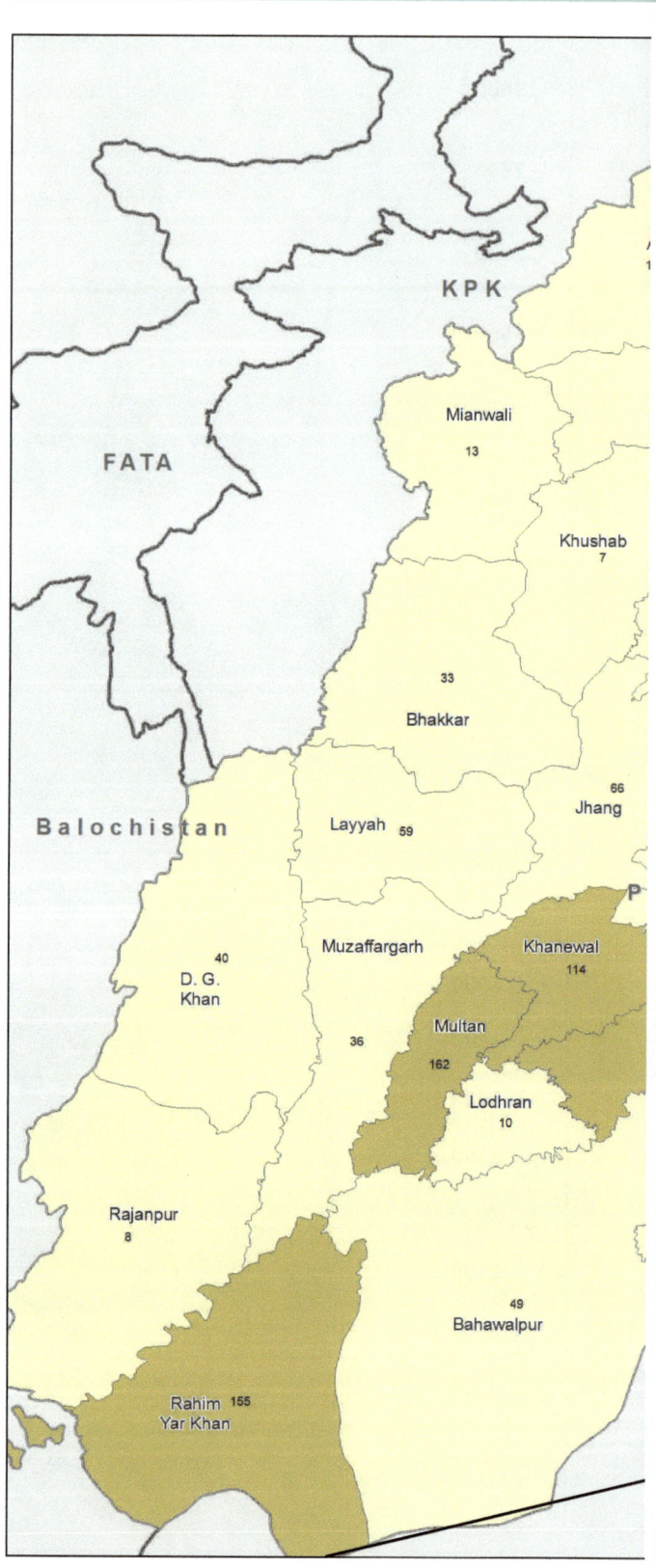

PUNJAB PROVINCE: Summary of Dengue fo

Legend

No. of Patients

	7 - 100
	101 - 200
	201 - 1000
	1001 - 17343

Provincial Boudray

District Boundary

Information Management Unit
Provincial Disaster Management Authority of Punjab

ever cases as of Nov. 15, 2011

Fig: 28

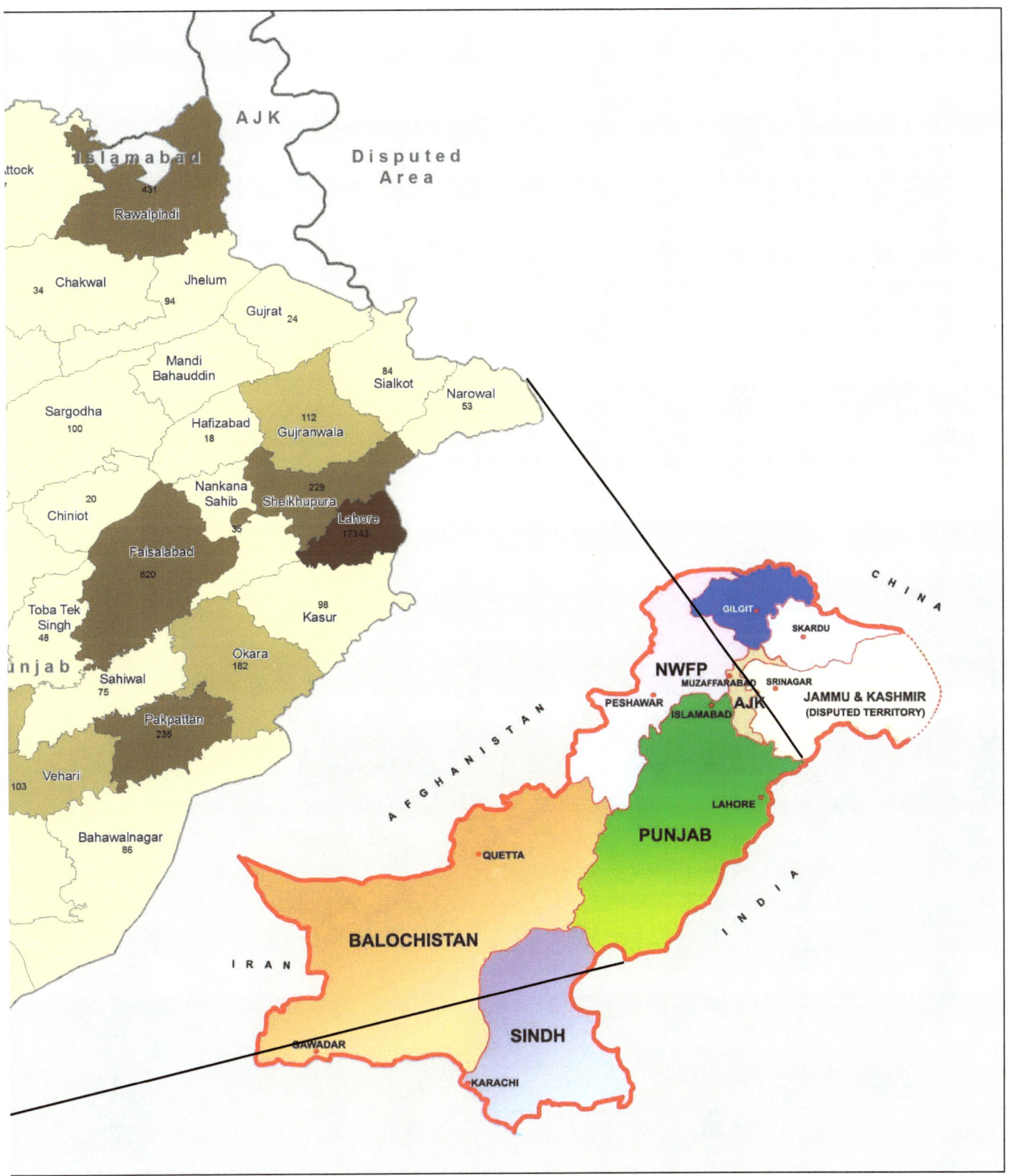

A J K

Islamabad

attock

431

Rawalpindi

Disputed
Area

34 Chakwal

Jhelum

94

Gujrat 24

Mandi
Bahauddin

84
Sialkot

Narowal
53

Sargodha
100

Hafizabad
18

112
Gujranwala

Chiniot

20

Nankana
Sahib

229
Sheikhupura

35

Lahore
17343

Faisalabad
820

Toba Tek
Singh
48

98
Kasur

unjab

Okara
182

Sahiwal
75

Pakpattan
235

Vehari

103

Bahawalnagar
86

C H I N A

GILGIT

SKARDU

NWFP

MUZAFFARABAD   SRINAGAR

PESHAWAR   AJK

ISLAMABAD

JAMMU & KASHMIR
(DISPUTED TERRITORY)

A F G H A N I S T A N

LAHORE

PUNJAB

QUETTA

I R A N

BALOCHISTAN

I N D I A

SINDH

GAWADAR

KARACHI

PROVINCIAL DISASTER MANAGEMENT AUTHORITY

To provide relief to the families of Dengue patients, Government of Punjab through PDMA, established six Relief Camps with the collaboration of Civil Defense (Table 1). These relief camps were established in six major hospitals of Lahore. One month's ration hampers were also supplied to Dengue patients admitted in these hospitals.

The officers of Civil Defense were engaged to ensure efficient and timely disbursement of relief packages offered by the provincial government. The Civil Defense also extended their cooperation in the process of documentation and verification of Dengue patients' families.

Establishment of Relief Camps — *Table: 1*

No.	Hospital Name	Food Hampers delivered
1	General Hospital	500
2	Mayo Hospital	491
3	Children Hospital	198
4	Ghanga Ram Hospital	200
5	Service Hospital	200
6	Jinnah Hospital	397
	Total	**1,986**

Wife of a Dengue patient receives food hamper — *Fig. 29*

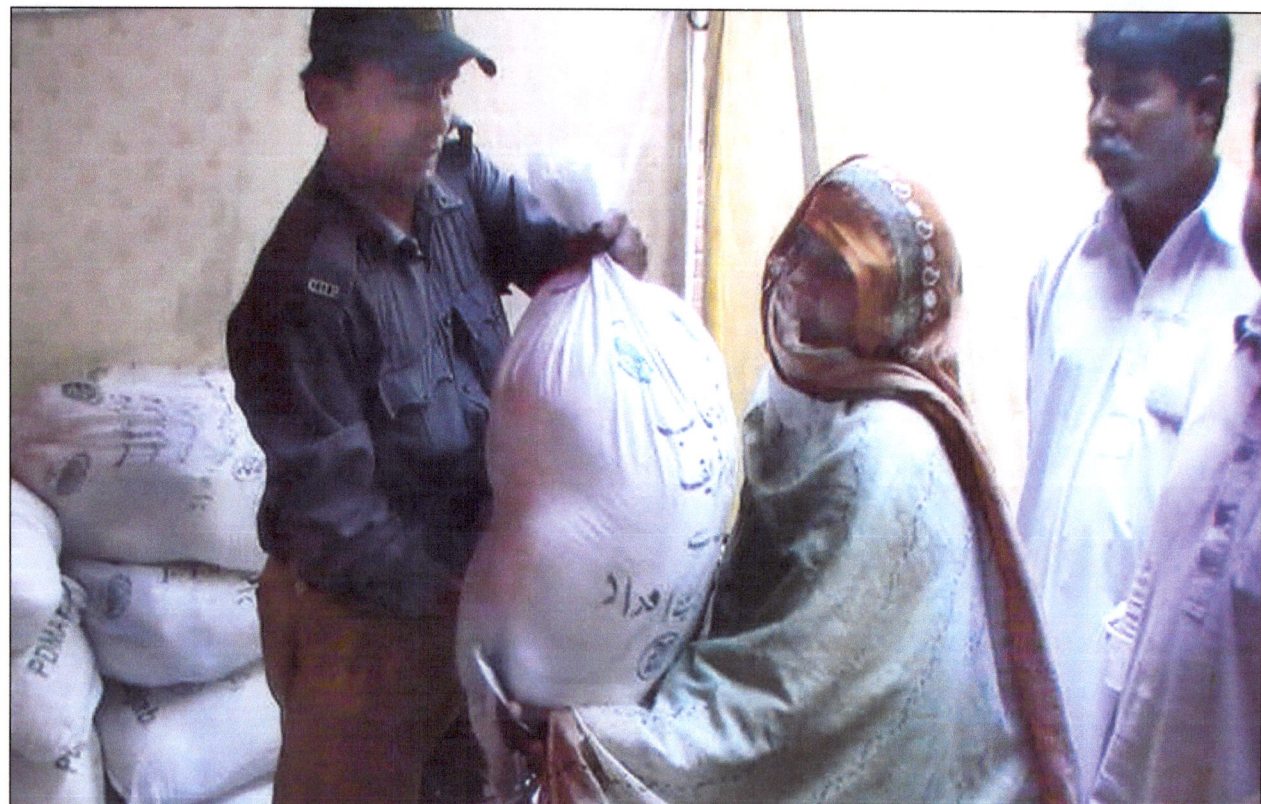

Airconditioned Field Hospitals and Relief Camps setup by PDMA   *Fig. 30*

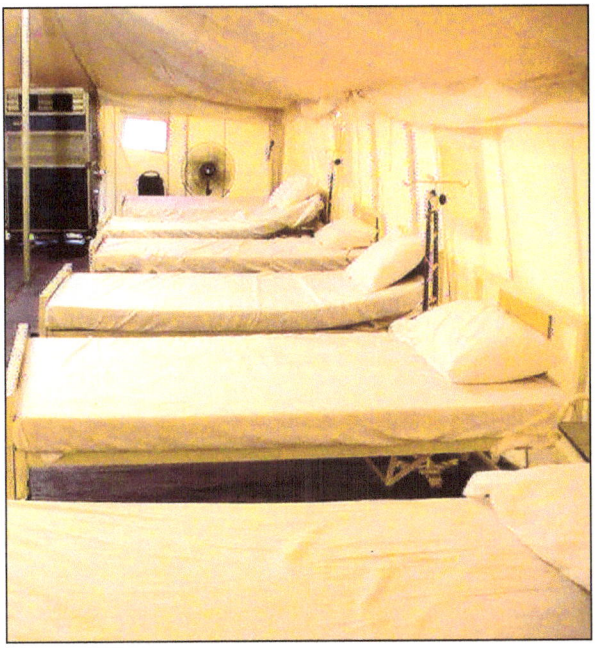

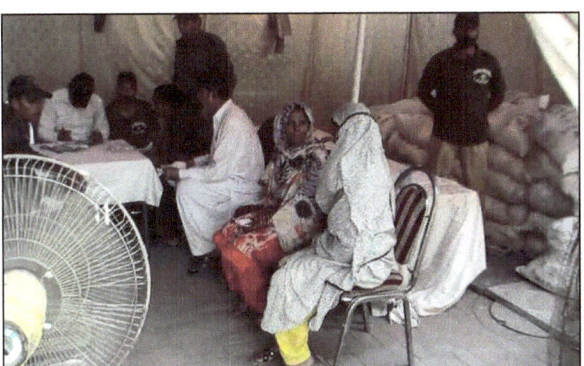

Establishment of Field Hospitals

The monsoon season saw a rapid influx of Dengue patients in the major hospitals of Lahore. Many of those patients had to be hospitalized to ensure their timely recovery. As the number of patients grew, the hospital resources came under severe constraint.

The large number of indoor patients left little room for the incoming Dengue patients that had to be hospitalized. To overcome this shortage, PDMA decided to setup eight field hospitals in the premises of six different government hospitals. These field hospitals were equipped with advanced health care facilities. An air conditioning system had also been installed to keep the internal environment at an optimal temperature.

These types of contingency arrangements prevented any mismanagement of Dengue patients who flocked to governmental facilities in large numbers when the epidemic outbreak reached its peak. It also showed that Government had planned in advance and was prepared to combat any extreme eventuality.

Documentation process for deserving patients   *Fig. 31*

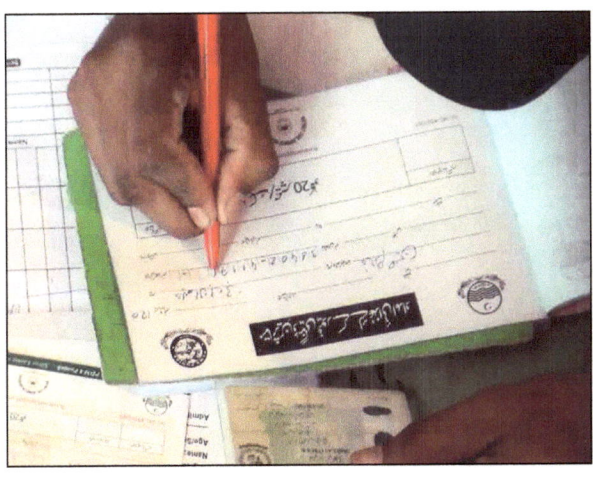

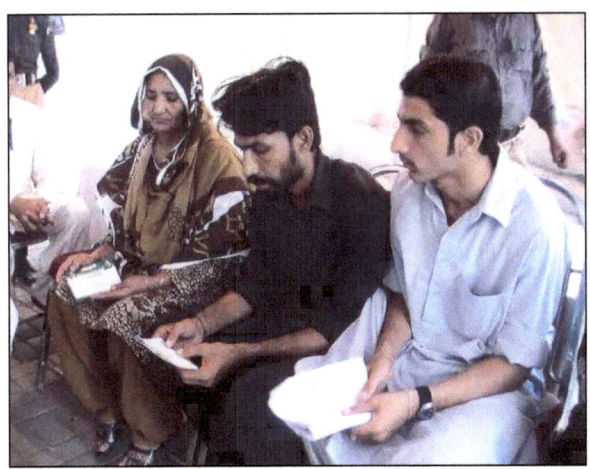

The Health Department collected data from all health facilities to implement the vector control program. The Department employed comprehensive disease surveillance tools to compile the data on Dengue cases. The comprehensive data was then divided on the basis of patient's addresses and was provided to the TMAs so that they could conduct chemical control in areas that were generating a large number of Dengue patients. Disease surveillance is an integral part of public health measures. The data on patients was received from all major hospitals of Punjab and was compiled and examined for analysis and segregation. The department also carried out health education activities, informing the public on the symptoms of Dengue fever and the measures that should be taken in case those symptoms are observed. Health education activities were carried out through print and electronic media, seminars and by mobilizing the Lady Health Workers. All the administrative units were monitored by Health Department to check larvicidal activity, fumigation and fogging in the districts. These activities were carried out with the help from district gov-

ernment. Health personnel from the Directorate General of Health Services were deputed for continuous monitoring of the chemical control. The Health Department was also directly involved in building the capacity of towns and districts to conduct a powerful chemical control, utilizing fogger sprays, insecticides, etc.

Strategy to Combat Dengue

Dengue is a fairly new phenomenon in Pakistan as shown in Figure 33 It was only in year 2011 that the epidemic reached unprecedented levels. That year the Health Department was involved in all aspects of the combat against Dengue fever. The department collaborated in the vector control efforts and mobilized the community through mass media, seminars, posters and leaflets etc. It provided additional Human Resources to the hospitals that saw a large influx of Dengue patients. It also provided additional equipment for the diagnostic center, and screening camps etc. The department sought to improve the clinical management in all health facilities which eventually reduced the mortalities.

A view of Dengue patients ward in a hospital Fig. 32

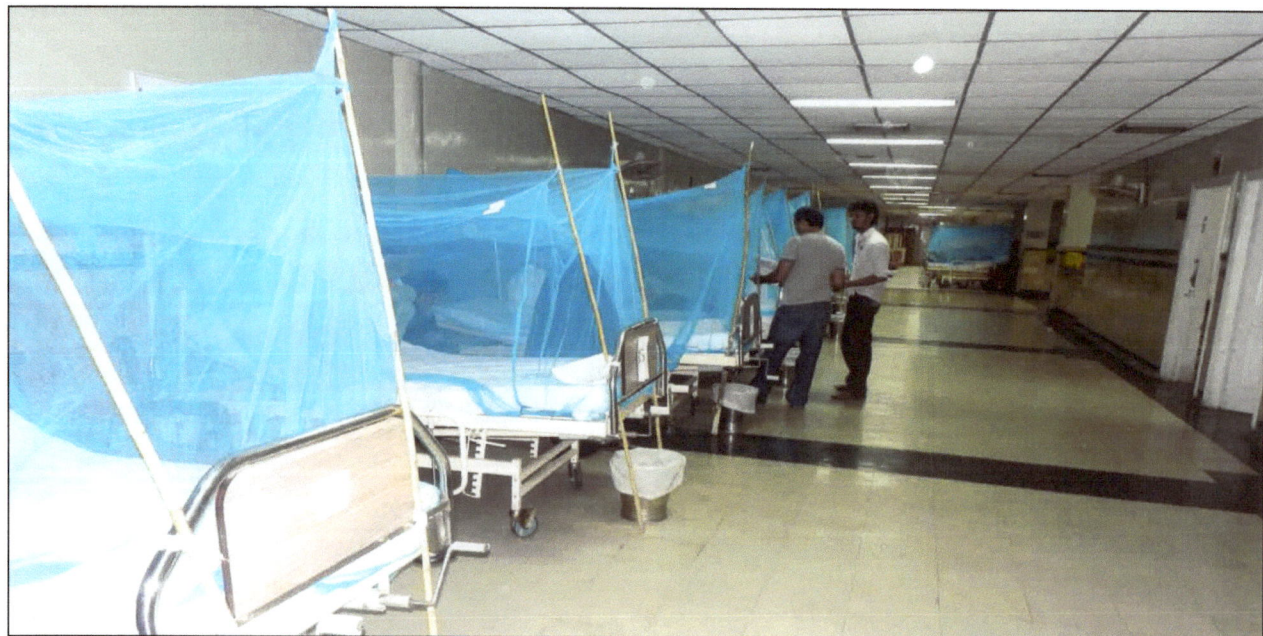

Yearly pattern of disease in Punjab *Fig. 33*

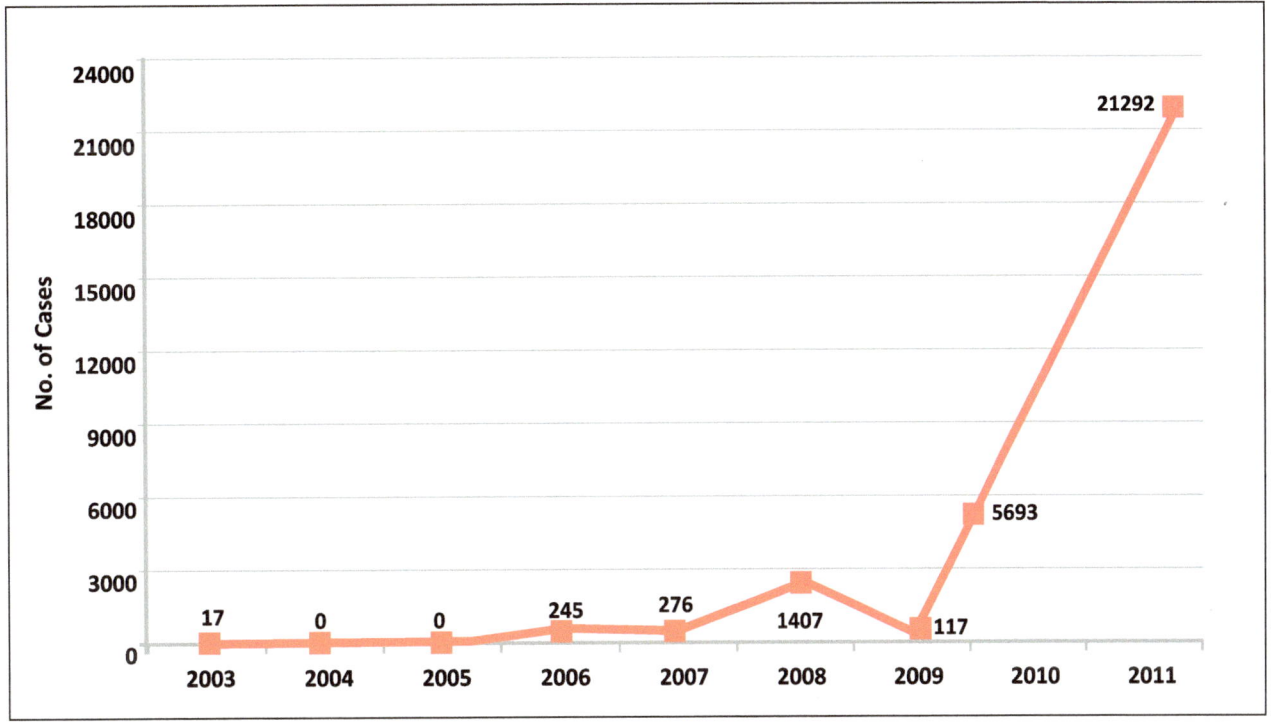

Paramedic staff attending Dengue patients *Fig. 34*

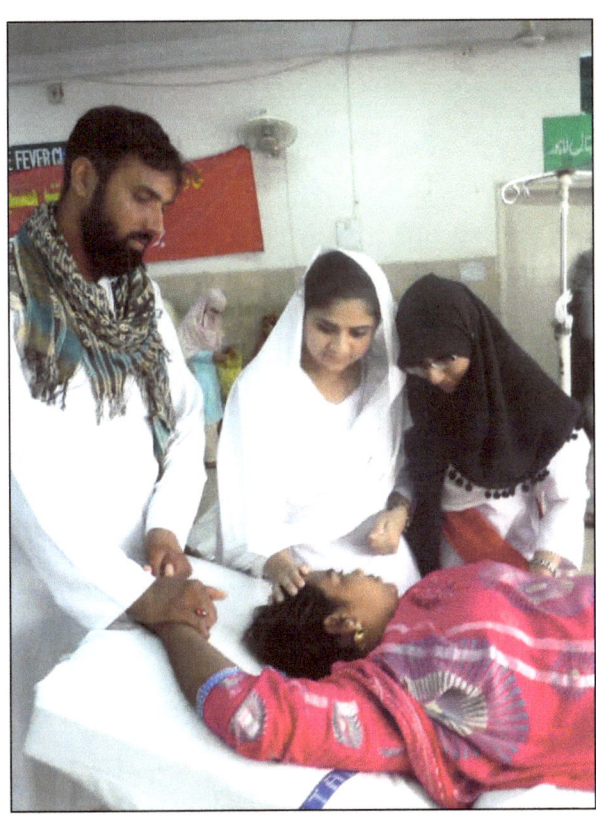
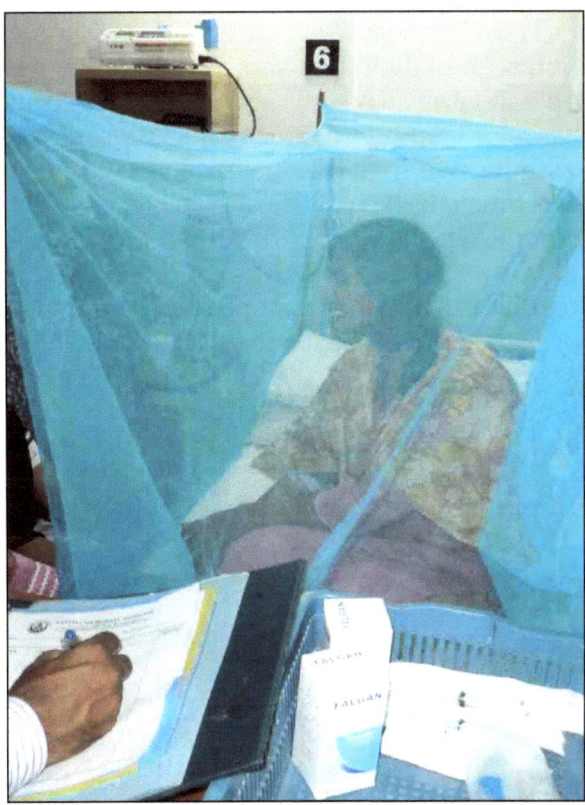

No.	Name of Hospital	No. of Beds specifically reserved for Dengue Patients
	Beds reserved for Dengue patients in major Private Hospitals of Lahore *Table: 2*	
1	Surraya Azeem Hospital	10
2	Surgimed Hospital	20
3	Ammar Medical Complex	10
4	Fatima Memorial	30
5	Shalimar Hospital	40
6	Family Hospital	10
7	Ghurki Hospital	30
8	Farooq Hospital	15
9	Ittefaq Hospital	Complete free treatment for Dengue patients
10	Hijaz Hospital	Complete free treatment for Dengue patients
	These hospitals also provided free OPD services	

Policy Guidelines

The Government of Punjab directed all private hospitals to dedicate special Dengue wards and reserve a certain percentage of beds for Dengue patients. Table 2 shows sample data of ten such private hospitals.

The administrators facing a risk of Dengue outbreak in their area should ensure proper operations in all health facilities. All suspected cases of Dengue fever should be provided with the necessary health care in a courteous and timely fashion. All health facilities should compile and report the data on patients. The data on patients should be analyzed on a regular basis so that any spike in the number of patients could be identified before the disease spreads any further. Proper supplies of medication and testing equipment should also be ensured. The administrators should

Established Dengue Ward *Fig. 35*

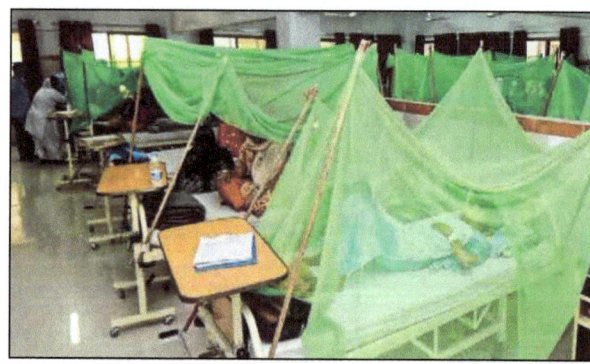

also carry out health education activities, informing the public on the symptoms of Dengue fever and the measures that should be taken in that case.

Table 3 shows the Proforma that should be filled by hospitals and testing centers for each patient with a positive test of Dengue fever.

No.	Case Report Date	Name of Patient	Sex	Age	Mohala	Tehsil & District	Contact No.	Name of Hospital / Lab.	Status	Lab. Result
	Proforma for the collection of patient information *Table: 3*									

Vector control is the primary responsibility of the City District Government. Vector control can be divded into chemical control, habitat or mechanical control, contact control, and biological control. Lahore is administratively divided into nine towns which are then further divided into a total of about 150 Union Councils (UC), as reflected in Table 4. The chemical control had been devolved to the town level. Town Municipal Officers (TMOs) created and mobilized teams of individuals responsible for fogging, Internal Residual Sprays (IRS) and larviciding. Chemical control formed the bulk of Government of Punjab's vector control programs as the vector colonies had already proliferated to the entire city when the Government initiated its response. The foremost priority of the City District Government of Lahore (CDGL) was to eradicate the source of this disease through fumigation. Throughout the chemical control campaign the CDGL was also working on other methods of vector control.

Chemical Control

Chemical control can be further divided into fogging, IRS, and Larviciding activities. Fogging has an immediate knock down effect and is conducted against the wind at a speed of 5km/hr. IRS is conducted in indoor settings to restrict the growth and breeding of *Aedes* mosquitoes. Larviciding is conducted to eliminate the larvae and is done by adding 20ml of liquid temifoss to 10 liters of water. All towns of Lahore had 35 small man mounted foggers and one large vehicle mounted fogger. Each town was responsible for the clean-up of UCs that fall within that town. The TMA planned and executed the chemical control of every single UC. A house to house coverage was planned before the foggers embarked on the fumigation campaign. Fogger teams were organized and dispatched to ensure the comprehensive fumigation of the entire town. The Government of Punjab used Deltamethrin and other chemicals to eradicate the vector populations through fogging. The fogging formulation consists of 250ml of Deltamethrin for every ten litres of diesel. Table 5 shows a sample template for tracking record of fogging which was maintained throughout the season.

Demographics of Lahore — Table: 4

Area of the District	1,772 Km^2
Total Population	9.0 million
Total Towns	9 + Cantt
Union Councils	150

Sample template of Fogging Schedule maintained throughout the season — Table: 5

Town	No. of UC Covered	No. of UC to be Covered	No of UC Being Covered Daily	Date When Cycle will be completed
Data Gunj Baksh	12	1	1	2nd October
Gulberg	11	4	2	3rd October
Samanabad	15	4	4	2nd October
Iqbal Town	7	11	3	5th October
Nishter	13	5	3	3rd October
Ravi	6	11	3	5th October
Shalimar	9	2	2	2nd October
Aziz Bhatti	12	1	1	2nd October
Wahga	6	6	2	2nd October

Parks and Horticulture Authority (PHA) took significant steps to eradicate all breeding spots in major parks of Lahore. The monsoon rains had created various pockets of stangnant water that acted as ideal habitats for *Aedes* Mosquitoes. This department either drained the water from all ponds or filled them with sand. The debris was cleaned and general cleanliness of the parks was ensured. The grass was cut on a regular basis and the irrigation of all the vegetation was tightly controlled in order to avoid any accumulation of water.

PHA initiated a comprehensive vector control in all major parks of the city. Larvicides and Insecticides were applied to eradicate any existing colonies in these parks. Tables 6 and 7 show a sample template of vector control schedule.

In colleberation with the Forest Department, PHA also introduced Tilapia fish in the relatively larger ponds of the parks. PHA did not confine its efforts to the parks of Lahore, they also assisted other departments by providing key resources. Each Union Council was provided an additional staff member to help with the fogging of that area and nine staff members of PHA were also deployed to the nine towns of Lahore. PHA also established a Dengue Diagnostic Center in the Khurshid Park neighborhood of Lahore. PHA equipped this center with doctors, technicians, support staff and sophisticated apparatus such as the Hematology Analyzer.

PHA operates more than 140 plant nurseries throughout the city. All of these nurseries were visited on a daily basis to remove any stagnant water. Larvicides were introduced

Sample template of the dates at which the major Parks of Lahore were fumigated   *Table: 6*

No.	Date	Name of Park	Location
1	19.9.2011	Jillani Park	Jail Road
2	20.9.2011	Badshahi Mosque Park	Circular Garden
3	20.9.2011	Taxali Family Park	Circular Garden
4	20.9.2011	Bhatigate Park	Circular Garden
5	20.9.2011	Ali Park	Circular Garden
6	20.9.2011	Lohari & Morigate Park	Circular Garden
7	20.9.2011	Mochigate Park	Circular Garden
8	20.9.2011	Yakigate Park	Circular Garden
9	20.9.2011	Sheranwala Park	Circular Garden
10	20.9.2011	Mastigate Park Akbarigate Park	Circular Garden
11	20.9.2011	Main Park Wassanpura	Wassanpura
12	21.9.2011	P-Block Park	Sabzazar Scheme
13	21.9.2011	G-Block Park	Sabzazar Scheme
14	21.9.2011	Cricket Ground Doongi Ground	Samanabad
15	21.9.2011	A-Block Park	Sabzazar Scheme
16	21.9.2011	B-Block Park	Sabzazar Scheme
17	22.9.2011	Nasir Bagh	Upper Mall
18	22.9.2011	Nehru Park	Sant Nagar
19	22.9.2011	Farrukhabad Park	Shahdrah
20	22.9.2011	Match Factory Cricket Ground	Shahdrah

in water ponds and fogging was conducted in these nurseries on a weekly basis. All broken earthen pots were removed from the private nurseries. Stagnant water in the empty earthen pots was drained and leaking water pots were plugged to avoid any unwanted accumulation of water. All the Directors of the Horticulture Department were directed to submit a certificate claiming that they have personally visited the parks & green belts in their jurisdiction and have ensured the general cleanliness, removal of debris from both inside and around the Parks, Greenbelts, etc. An additional committee was also formed to monitor and evaluate the work of all Directors on a regular basis.

Summary of Fumigation in major Parks *Table: 7*

No.	Date	No. of Parks	Date	No. of Parks
1	20-Sep-11	10	21-Sep-11	22
2	22-Sep-11	04	23-Sep-11	13
3	24-Sep-11	11	25-Sep-11	11
4	26-Sep-11	09	27-Sep-11	05
5	28-Sep-11	14	29-Sep-11	08
6	30-Sep-11	10	01-Oct-11	11

Fumigation in major Parks *Fig. 36*

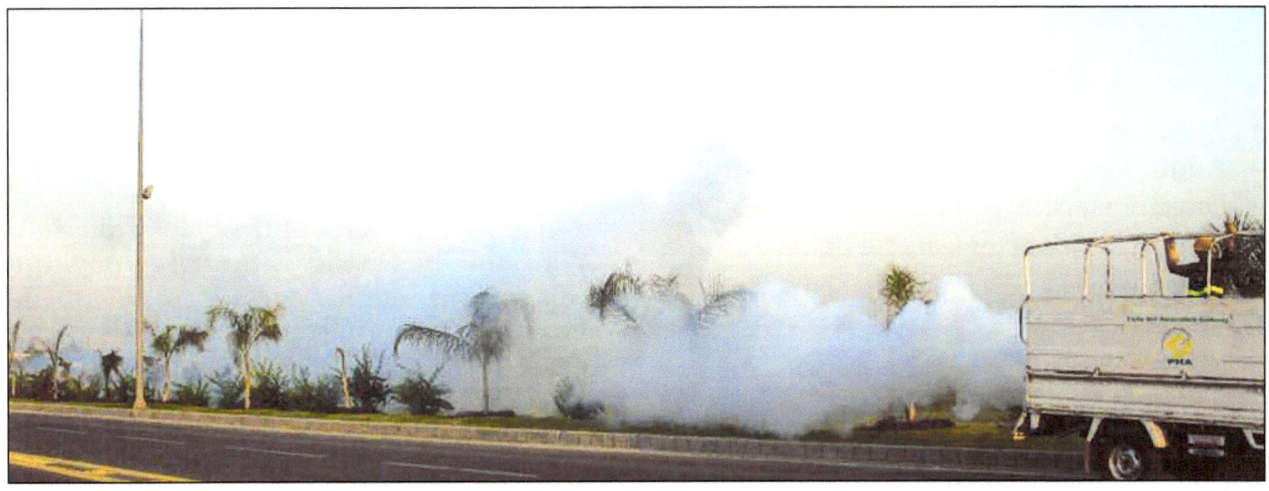

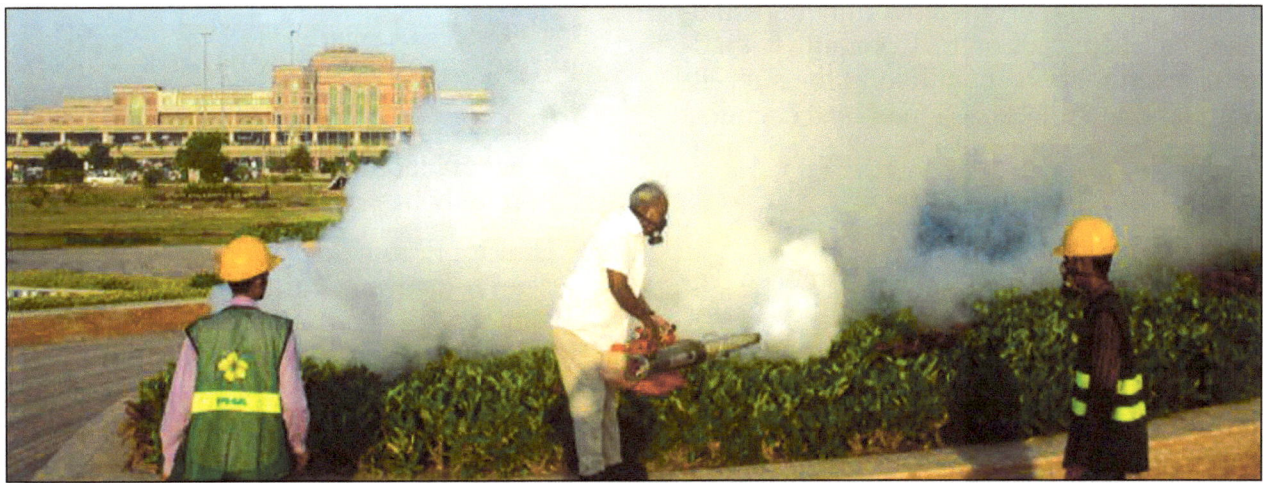

The Agriculture Department created a team of Entomologists to study the prevalence of larvae and adult mosquitoes.This study on prevalence gave the government a fair idea of areas that needed extensive chemical control. The Agriculture Department identified hot- spots that had large population of *Aedes* mosquitoes. These hot-spots were then communicated to TMAs so that they could conduct Fogging, IRS and Larviciding in those particular areas.

Surveillance Committee

Agriculture Department formulated a Surveillance Committee for Dengue control. This committee gave policy direction to the team of Entomologists and comprised of the following:

- A Member of National Assembly
- A Member of Provincial Assembly
- Secretary Agriculture Department
- Secretary Higher Education Department
- Additional Inspector General of Police
- Additional Secretary Higher Education
- Director General Agriculture Extension
- Additional Director General PHA
- Director Food

Terms of Reference

The Surveillance Committe developed Standard Operating Procedures for Surveillance, tapped the available expertise from within and beyond the government, established a Chemical Control Committe to eradicate the hot-spots identified in the surveillance and led the execution of post chemical control evaluation.

Obectives

Aedes mosquito population had been significantly increased due to continuous rains which resulted in high humidity and warm temperature. The surveillance of its burgeoning population was required to plan the chemical and non chemical control measures.

Strategy

Dedicated teams of the Entomologists were engaged for pest scouting to estimate the population of adults and larvae of *Aedes* mosquitoes. Ten teams of four persons each conducted sampling at ten sites daily. Each team member visited a specific geographically assigned location.

Operations

The following steps were undertaken by the Agriculture Department to ensure a city wide surveillance of *Aedes* mosquitoes.

• The Surveillance teams identified areas where larvae or adult mosquitoes were present. A Chemical Control team then eradicated the vector habitat from that area. A third team then conducted the post chemical control evaluation, and inspected the area that had been cleared by the chemical control

• Training on identification of adult, larvae and habitats was imparted to the field teams of Entomologists

• Assistant Director of the Plant Protection Wing and the District Officer of Agriculture (Extension) monitored at least 5% of the field reports through cross examination

• Field teams inspected all potential objects, habitats and breeding places identified by the experts. Their visits used to span over eight hours, starting from 7:30 am.

• The Control Room reported on spots requiring Chemical Control. District Government liaison officer ensured action on the spots and returned information listing the number of identified spots treated and pending on daily basis

• Director Entomology of Ayub Agricultural Research Institute, Faisalabad oversaw the execution of post chemical control evaluation of treated sites to assess the level of *Aedes* population. The DG of Agriculture (Extension) implemented this plan through field and data compilation teams

Progress of Surveillance Teams

Field teams generated surveillance reports of all nine towns of Lahore. The Food Department sent thirteen Officers to join this surveillance activity. The Pest Warning Wing of the Agriculture Department deployed additional Entomologists increasing the number to 71. The data compiled by the surveillance teams for Lahore served as a bench mark. These Entomologists conducted spot checks at about 12,000 places. Their surveillance helped the rest of the departments in narrowing their vector control efforts to the identified habitats.

Post Chemical Control Evaluation Teams

Post chemical control evaluation teams were mobilized to inspect whether there were still any larvae or mosquitoes left after fogging the areas where a vector had been observed earlier. Table 8 shows the sample template in which data was collected during the entire exercise.

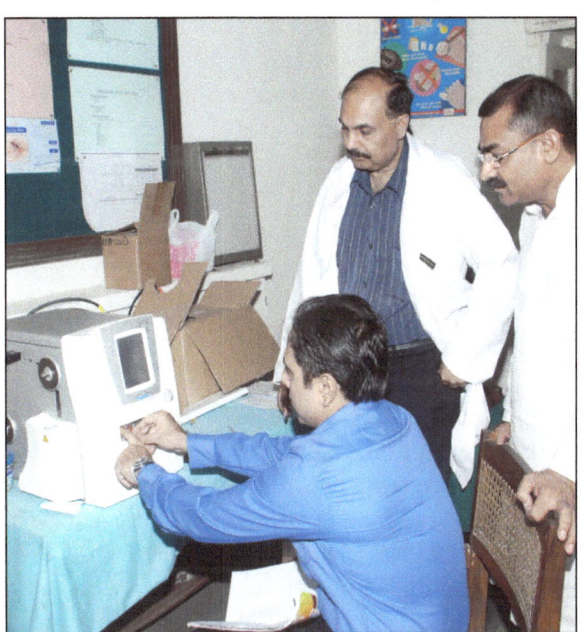

Surveillance Team   Fig. 37

Post Chemical Control Evaluation Data   Table: 8

No.	Date	Town	Spots Inspected	Larvae Prevalence	% Age	Adult Prevalence	% Age
1	25.09.2011	1	23	0	00.00	10	43.00
2	26.09.2011	7	85	14	16.47	29	34.11
3	27.09.2011	6	46	5	10.86	8	17.39
4	28.092011	10	53	2	03.77	12	22.64
5	29.09.2011	10	50	5	10.00	14	28.00
6	30.09.2011	10	38	8	21.05	9	23.68
7	01.10.2011	10	70	8	11.43	22	25.00
8	02.10.2011	10	58	12	20.69	19	32.75
	Total		423	54	12.76	123	29.70

Policy Guidelines

In case of an onset of this epidemic, the adminstrator of that area should create a Surveillance Committee consisting of key political and governmental figures. This committee should provide policy guidelines to a team of Entomologists which the adminstrator should nominate in coordination with the district representative of Agriculture Department. The surveillance team of Entomologists should then conduct spot-checks to study the presence of larvae or adult mosquitoes.

An analysis based on the data generated by Entomologists team would identify spots that need chemical control or fumigation due to high prevalence of larvae or adult mosquitoes. The team should recheck the same spot after chemical control to ensure its proper efficiency.

The team of Entomologists should conduct spot checks on a daily basis and fill the proforma in Table 9 to allow a comprehensive analysis of vector prevalence. Table 10 should be filled to collect the data on chemical control.

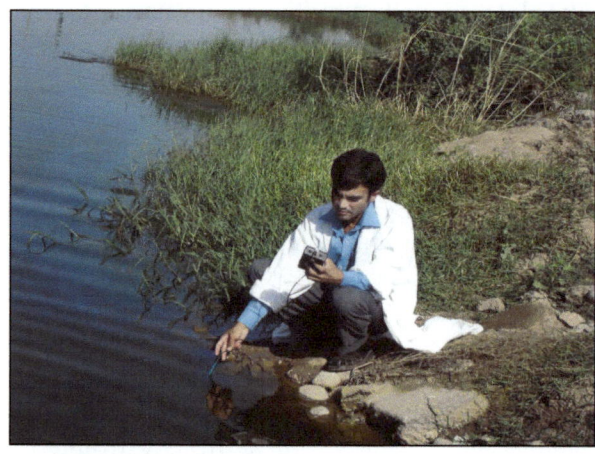

Entomologist conducting a spot-check *Fig.38*

Template for the collection of data on hot-spots *Table: 9*

No.	Date	Tehsil	Habitats Identified Proposed	Chemical and Postchemical control	Vector Prevalence

Additional template for the collection of data on hot-spots *Table: 10*

No.	Tehsil	Spots Inspected	Larvae Prevalence	%age Prevalence	Adult Prevalence	%age Prevalence

The Irrigation Department was called in help of the Health Department to provide extra Human Resources and I.T. facilities. It was responsible for the monitoring and evaluation of the medical services that were provided to the patients of Dengue fever.

Table 11 shows a sample template providing a comprehensive overview of the level of services which were provided at all of the major hospitals of Lahore. This data was updated daily by the Irrigation Department. A Short Messaging System (SMS) based facility was used in which each hospital was visited by an Irrigation Department employee, who reported data of Table 11 through cell phone.

Overview of the treatment provided at the hospitals of Lahore   *Table: 11*

No.	Name of Hospital	Total Beds in Hospital	Total Beds for Dengue Patients	Total Dengue Patients Admitted	Total No. of Free Patients Admitted	Total Beds for Dengue Patients	Platelets Bottle Required	Status of Treatements
1	Adil Hospital	50	15	4	7	8	0	Satisfactory
2	Akhtar Saeed Trust Hosepitall	300	40	6	19	21	0	Good
3	Akram Medical Complex	25	5	2	5	0	0	Good
4	Al-Ehsanl Hospital	62	62	55	55	7	0	Good
5	Al-Shafi Hospital	13	3	2	0	1	0	Bad
6	Ammar Medical Complex	30	10	5	8	2	0	V.Good
7	Arif Memorial Teaching Hospital	400	40	2	14	26	0	Good
8	Bahria Town Hospital	50	15	2	11	4	0	Good
9	Bajwa Hospital Shahdra	30	10	8	8	4	0	Bad
10	Cardex Medical Centre	40	10	0	2	8	0	Good
11	Cavalry Hospital	17	4	2	2	2	0	Satisfactory
12	Ch. Rehmat Memorial Trust Hospital	300	70	10	38	32	0	Good
13	Doctors Hospital	112	18	4	8	14	0	Good
14	Family Hospital	45	8	26	5	2	0	Satisfactory
15	Farooq Hospital	70	40	34	6	9	0	V.Good
16	Fatima Memorial Hospital	540	60	4	40	20	0	Good
17	Fauji Foundation	170	40	40	32	0	0	Satisfactory
18	Fazal Hospital	18	5	5	0	0	0	Good
19	Ghurki Trust Hospital	450	15	43	15	0	0	Good
20	Hameed Latif Hospital	200	50	36	7	14	0	V.Good
21	Hijaz Hospital	60	17	5	5	12	0	Good
22	Ihsan Mumtaz Hospital	15	2	1	1	1	0	Satisfactory
23	Iqra Medical Complex	30	7	6	6	1	0	Good
24	Ittefaq Hospital	435	90	26	90	0	0	Excellent
25	Jamiyyat Hospital	11	4	6	6	0	0	Good
26	Khair-un-Nisa Hospital	40	10	1	1	9	0	Satisfactory
27	Mansoora Hospital	150	20	7	25	0	0	V.Good
28	Masood Hospital	20	5	4	4	1	0	Good
29	Mumtaz Bakhtawar Hospital	100	60	20	20	40	0	Excellent
30	Naseer Hospital Garden Town	20	6	0	2	4	0	Good

The Auqaf and Religious Affairs Department deals with shrines and other religious institutions. It engaged religious Scholars and Madrassas (religious schools) in a public awareness campaign. Ulema (religious leaders) across the region were communicated on the disastrous impacts of an epidemic outbreak and were engaged to communicate the importance of Dengue prevention. Ulema command a wide audience which is willing to follow their suggestions. Ulema raised the awareness of masses at large religious gatherings such as Friday prayers. The Auqaf Department also created a partnership with different Madrassas to raise awareness through their students.

Action Plan

1. In compliance with the instructions of the Chief Minister Punjab, Auqaf & Religious Affairs Department launched a campaign against Dengue virus at various levels through Ulema, Mashaikh and other Religious Scholars in Mosques, Shrines and Madrassas

2. An "Emergency Community Mobilization Committee for Dengue Control Campaign" headed by a member of National Assembly was constituted. The Secretary of Auqaf & Religious Affairs Department was also a senior member of the committee. The department prepared an action plan to launch community mobilization campaign. Broad outline of the action plan is as under:

- Engage Ulema in the public awareness campaign to reach large audiences during prayer times especially the Friday prayers

- Develop partnership with Madrassas in order to spread the message through students and teachers

- Involve members of Ittehaad Bain-ul-Muslamin (Unity for Muslims) for a joint declaration addressed to public at large

- Mass awareness through TV Talk Shows by Ulema

- Mobilize Ulema teams for visits to mosques throughout the city and to distribute published material to the public.

3. The following steps were taken by the Religious Affairs department in their Anti-Dengue campaign:

- A meeting of Ulema with the Chief Minister was held to mobilize them in a comprehensive Public Awareness Campaign

- Anti-Dengue Awareness Campaign was launched from Badshahi Mosque. Printed material especially pamphlets for Anti-Dengue campaign were disseminated to the general public

- Razakars (volunteers) at the Shrine of Hazrat Data Ganj Baksh (RA) were engaged in the campaign against Dengue. A cleanliness operation was carried out and pamphlets on Dengue prevention were distributed

- Three seminars were held for Dengue prevention in various shrines

- The Department conducted awareness campaign at Jamia Ashrafia, at Jamia Naeemia and at Australia Mosque. The Ulema addressed the audience and provided information for awareness to take preventive measures against Dengue Virus.

- A meeting of members of Ittehaad Bain-ul-Muslamin was held and a joint declaration for commitment to fight against Dengue was issued collectively. The meeting was widely advertised through print and electronic media.

- A meeting of Religious Scholars was organized by Jamiat Ahal-Hadis and a Dengue Prevention Seminar was conducted at Badshahi Mosque.

- The officers of Auqaf & Religious Affairs Department visited three Madrassas and provided informative material on Dengue prevention.

- A special meeting of Ittehaad Tanzimaat Deenia was held where a joint declaration was made to organize awareness campaign amongst the students and teachers of Madrassas regarding the Dengue Virus.

- Madrassas for girl students were engaged for creating public awareness through Idara Minhaj-ul-Hussain.

- CDs of documentary movie and printed material on prevention of the disease were delivered to the students of Madrassas. TV Talk Shows of Ulema were also organized to spread the knowledge on Dengue.

- Twelve teams of Ulema comprising of four members each were constituted to visit mosques in Lahore. Seven hundred and twenty-nine mosques were visited by the Auqaf teams and all mosque incharges were informed of the Dengue related instructions. The pamphlets prepared by the Govt of Punjab were circulated amongst these participants.

- A 25 bed Dengue Ward was especially established at Data Darbar Hospital. All the laboratory tests and medicines were free of charge for all the patients. Doctors alongwith paramedical staff remained available around the clock.

Policy Guidelines

The adminstrator facing a risk of Dengue epidemic should engage religious Scholars and Madarassas in public awareness campaigns. Ulema across the district can communicate on the disastrous impacts of an epidemic outbreak. They can also communicate the mechanical controls through which the residents of districts can eliminate potential breeding spots of *Aedes* mosquitoes.

Anti-Dengue campaign launched from Badshahi Mosque *Fig. 39*

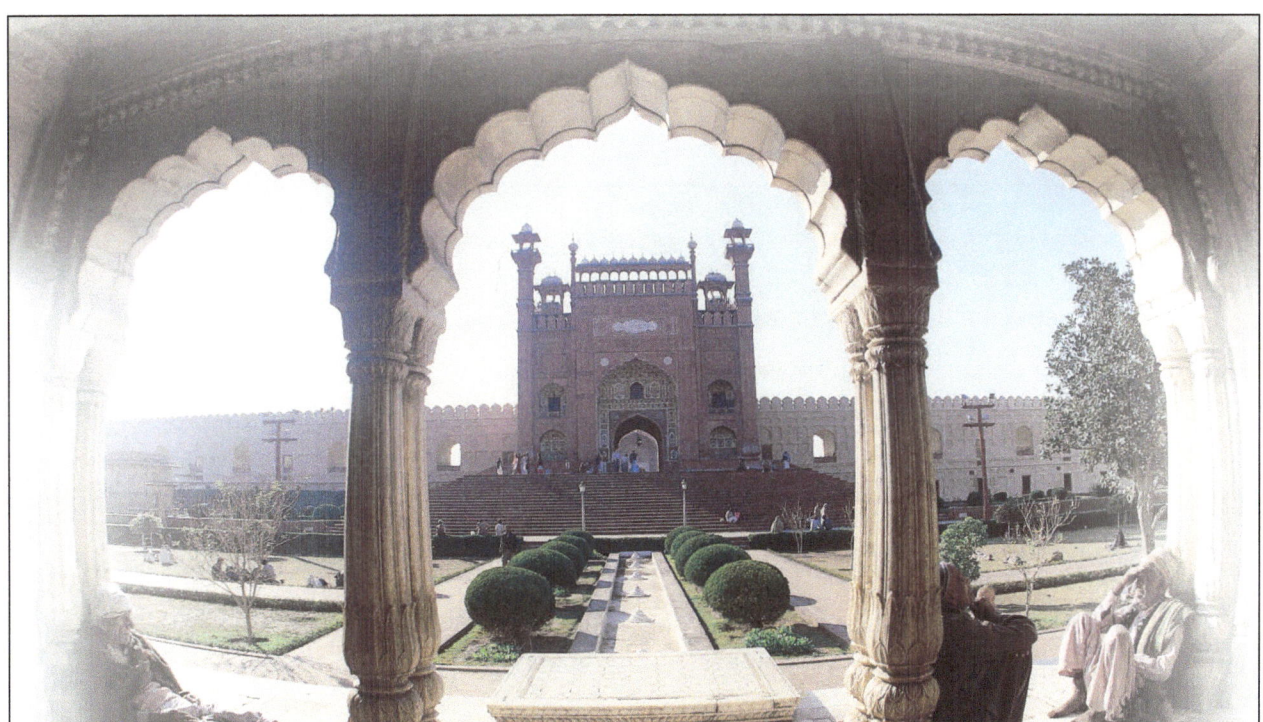

There are a total of 127 housing societies in Lahore, 70 of which are functional, and 57 are uninhabited at this point in time. The objective of Coopearatives Department was to undertake all possible actions for the prevention of Dengue fever by encouraging the housing societies to conduct Thermal Spray / Fumigation, IRS, Larviciding, cleanliness drives, and awareness campaigns for the prevention of Dengue fever. Table 12 shows a sample template of these operations in selected housing colonies.

The Cooperatives Department controls the various housing societies which are managed by various citizen-led cooperative societies The Cooperatives Department initiated a comprehensive cleanliness drive with the help of different housing societies of Lahore. The department created 17 monitoring teams that evaluated the cleanliness and chemical control operations of the housing societies of Lahore. The monitoring teams reported on the levels of cleanliness on a daily basis. The Cooperatives Department also arranged training workshops for the members & staff of the cooperative societies.

Information and educational communcation material was disseminated to all key stake holders in the management committees of the various housing societies of Lahore. Training workshops were conducted for the members/staff of the cooperative societies.

Action Plan

Following steps were taken to combat Dengue in the housing colonies

- Awareness campaigning through display of banners, distribution of leaflets and affixing Posters/Panaflexes
- Comprehensive cleanliness operations including removal of solid waste, garbage, debris and de-watering/drying of open spaces
- Involvement of public and private institutions for optimum resource utilization

Larviciding in a housing society *Fig. 40*

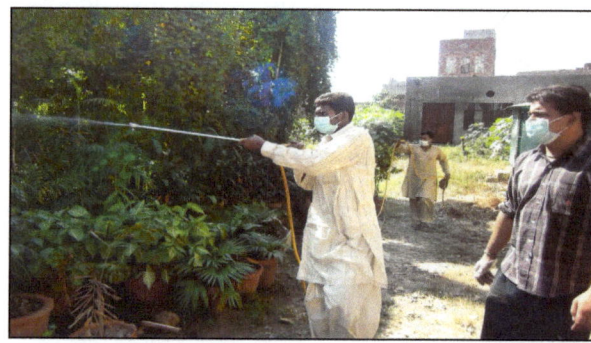

Sample template of monitoring visits conducted the Cooperatives Department *Table: 12*

No.	Name of Societies	Cleanliness	Thermal Fogging	Indoor Residual Spray (IRS)	Larvicide preventive measures
1	Government Employees Cooperative Housing Society (Phase-I), Township, Lahore	Good	Yes	Yes	Yes
2	Government Employees Cooperative Housing Society Link Model Town Road, Lahore.	Good	Yes	Yes	Yes
3	Gosha-e-Ahbab Cooperative Housing Society, Multan Road, Lahore	Un-Satisfactory	Yes	Yes	Yes
4	WAPDA Town Cooperative Housing Society (Phase-II)	Un-Satisfactory	Yes	Yes	Yes

Policy Guidelines

The administrators facing an epidemic outbreak should insure that the housing societies in their jurisdiction are clean and free of water ponds. Regularly cleaned and well maintained housing societies do not offer favorable breeding spots for *Aedes* mosquitoes. The administrators should create a monitoring team that evaluates the levels of cleanliness and chemical control operations at the different housing societies of that area.

Table 13 shows a sample proforma which can be used to keep track of the coordination with the teams responsible for ensuring clean and healthy housing societies.

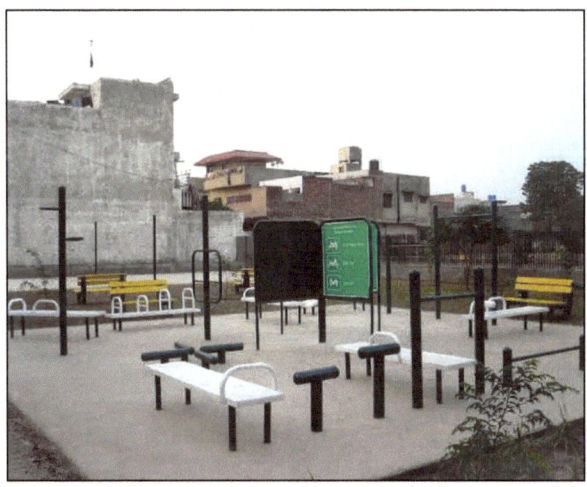
A cleaned park in a housing society — Fig. 41

Sample template for keeping track of coordination with teams — Table: 13

No.	Name of Societies	Cleanliness	Thermal fogging	Internal Residual Spray	Larvaciding

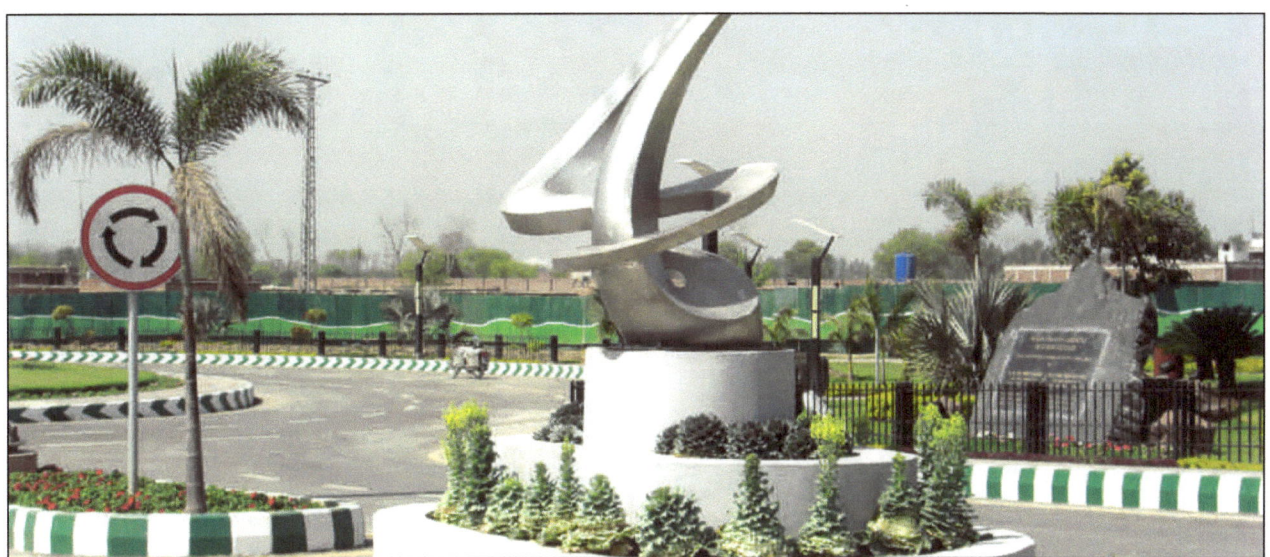
View of a cleaned Housing Society after a massive cleaning operation — Fig. 42

A Central Emergency Response Committee (CERC) was formed to meet on a regular basis to streamline the efforts of all departments of the Government of Punjab. The CERC was chaired by MNA Hamza Shahbaz Sharif. This Committee coordinated the departmental efforts and provided overall guidance on Dengue prevention and control. It routinely took macro and microlevel decisions and requested compliance progress from other departments on them. Table 14 gives examples of the decisions that were taken by this committee and the progress that was reported back.

Sample template of decisions taken by CERC *Table: 14*

No.	Decision	Progress
1	Facilities of cell separator at Institute of Blood Transfusion Lahore are inadequate. Cell separator machines at private hospitals i.e. Sheikh Zayed hospital Lahore, Air Force hospital, CMH, etc. may be integrated with the public sector effort to facilitate general public	Institute of blood transfusion was visited and five Cell Separators were arranged on placement basis in collaboration with Hospital Supply Corporation (Pvt)
2	Information of Cell Separation facilities at Call Center Helpline should be available	The list of private facilities was provided to the Helpline
3	Procurement of (CBC) Analyzer must be expedited	A short tender notice was issued and CBC analyzers were delivered within 3 weeks
4	Private medical colleges and allied teaching hospitals to reserve free beds for Dengue as per the requirement of PDMC	100% free accommodation and consultation was provided, as per the requirements of PDMC
5	Ten Diagnostic Camps to be made operational	Ten Diagnostic Camps in partnership with Chughtai Lab were made operational

Meeting of CERC chaired by MNA. Hamza Shahbaz Sharif *Fig. 42*

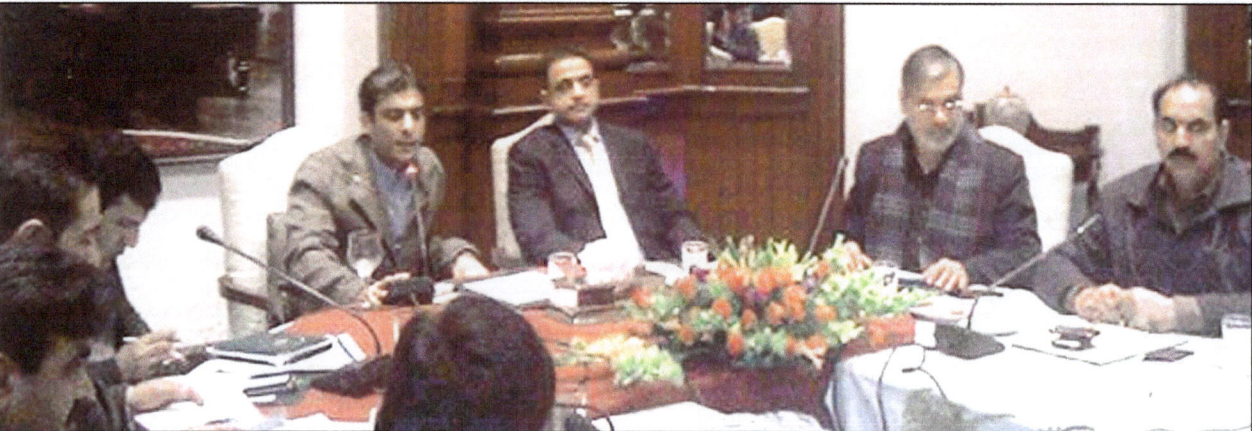

No.	Decision	Progress
6	Assistance to Cantonment General Hospital Lahore	EDO (H) Lahore visited the hospital in compliance with the instruction
7	Scare created by mosquito repellant and insecticide companies in their advertisements may be rectified	Secretary IT Department coordinated with chairman PEMRA to make necessary revisions in the advertisements
8	Psychiatrist and psychologist should be provided for patient counseling	Psychiatrists and psychologists were regularly visiting hospitals for counseling of patients and their attendants
9	Establishment of 30 Counseling Camps	Counseling camps had been established
10	NGO's linkage in Dengue prevention and control	Meeting with representatives of 65 NGOs was held on 12-09-2011 at 02:00 pm.
11	Facilitation to visiting Sri Lankan medical team	DG Protocol and DGHS provided all possible assistance to the medical team
12	Press briefing of Dengue	A press conference was held by the Health Advisor Mr. Khawaja Salman Rafiq
13	Private hospitals be integrated in Dengue control and management campaign and beds be reserved for Dengue patients, free of charge	The private hospitals unanimously agreed to provide free diagnostic services and 165 beds for Dengue patients
14	Weakness in IRS strategy may be removed and it may be decentralized to Towns	Town-wise information was communicated to town emergency response committees for focused IRS campaign. The Dean of IPH monitored and validated the IRS activity
15	Helpline to be made fully functional	Helpline was kept fully functional
16	School / Higher Education Department to step up efforts for awareness	The Departments conducted seminars in schools and colleges
17	Sheikh Zayed Hospital to provide full cover for dengue cases. A separate dengue ward be established	Instruction issued to CEO of Sheikh Zayed Hospital Lahore
18	Additional Support to be provided to DHA for Larviciding activities	Action taken by DCO Lahore
19	Provision of two additional Blood Analyzers for Ganga Ram Hospital, Lahore	Two Blood Analyzers were installed within a week's time

The Environment Department conducted a tyre management campaign to dispose the tyres that could act as potential habitats for *Aedes* Mosquitoes. Tyre markets were visited to inspect the prevalence of vector. The department treated and relocated almost all tyres that were stored in the open. Tyres act as womb for mosquitoes. Typically stored and stacked up in open, they accumulate rain water and become perfect humid breeding grounds for mosquitoes. Apart from tyres, the department also took care of natural breeding spots such as tree holes, water coolers, etc.

Removal of Vector Habitats

The Environment Department worked on the removal of vector habitats. They sought to eradicate the ideal breeding sites such as tyres, broken ceramic-ware, tree holes and water coolers. The water accumulated in the waste lying in open can pose a significant threat to the health of nearby communities. Environment Department helped in the removal of waste and debris. The stagnant water from tree holes or roadside puddles was drained. These governmental efforts had to be supported by the cooperation of the communities. The residents of Lahore had to be sensitized to the importance of taking similar measures at the household level.

The Environmental Protection Agency conducted a massive awareness campaign to get the citizens involved in the vector control. This awareness campaign involved the following actions:

• Seminars and Workshops

• Disbursement of Pamphlets, Brochures and Charts.

• Awareness Walks

• Establishment of Environment Clubs in Schools.

Tyre Management Campaign

The Environment Department undertook the greatest tyre-centric vector control in the world. Almost no tyre was left in the open. A Chief Minister's special committee for tyre management was setup. The objective of this committee was to oversee the enforcement of rules regarding proper management of used tyres. Used tyres are the single most important source of vector breeding. Tyre markets, godowns and open junk yards were inspected in large numbers and those which did not comply had to face legal repercussions.

Environment Department's intervention at Tyre warehouses Fig. 44

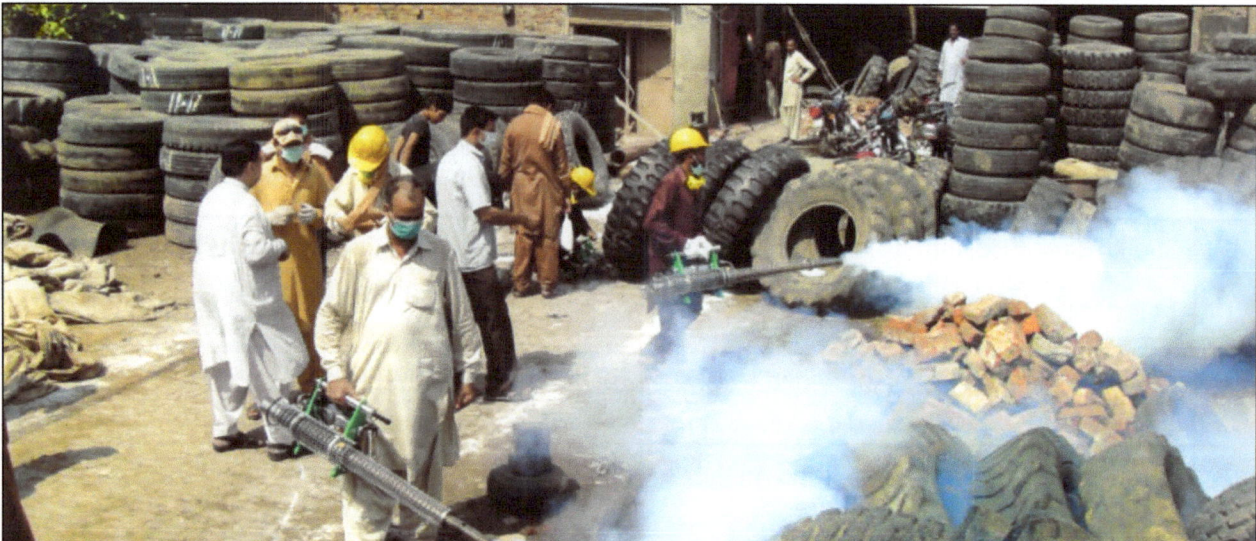

Policy Guidelines

The administrators for a particular region should ensure that all possible habitats of *Aedes* mosquitoes are eliminated. A comprehensive tyre management campaign should be undertaken to treat and relocate the tyres that are stored in the open. Apart from tyres, the administrators must also take care of natural breeding spots such as tree holes water containers, etc. The presence of vector should be reinspected after the removal of such potential habitats.

Parliamentarians at a Tyre warehouses *Fig. 45*

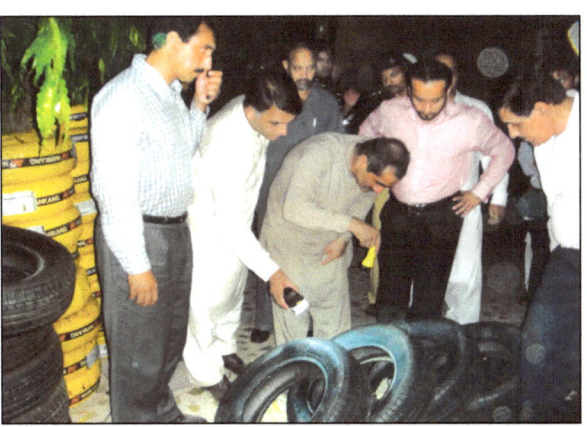

Larva surveillance at various Tyre warehouses *Fig. 46*

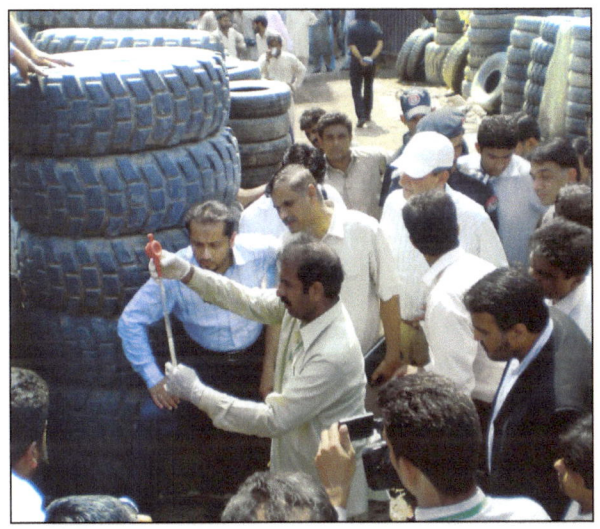
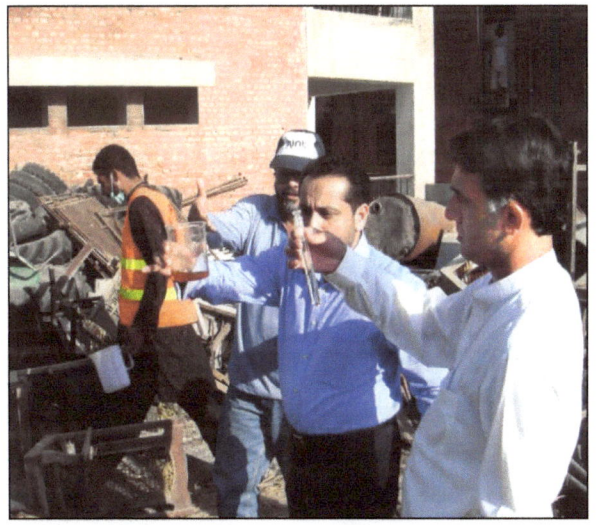
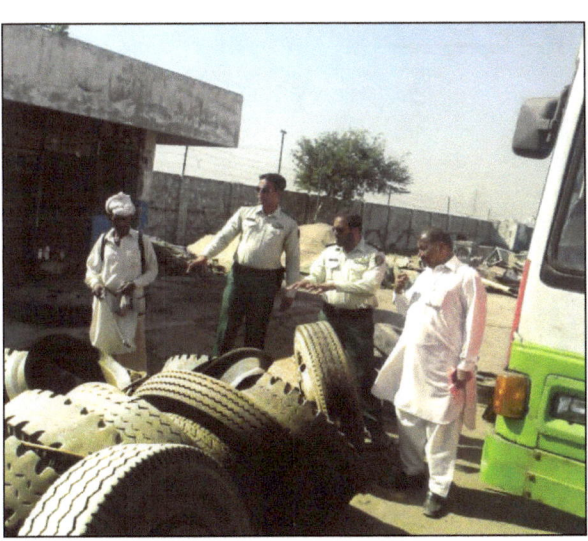
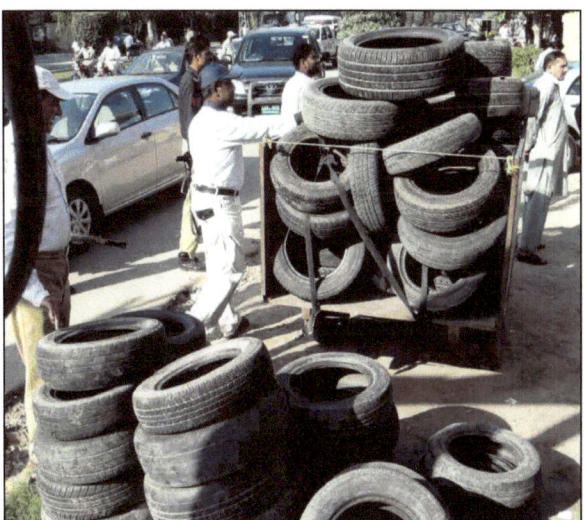

The Forests and Fisheries Department planned and implemented a biological control program utilizing fish that feed on larvae. The department cultured Tilapia, Grass Carp and Gambusia in controlled settings and then introduced them to ponds where *Aedes* mosquitoes could lay their eggs. The district officers for fisheries were trained to introduce this fish in water ponds that can serve as egg-laying areas for the *Aedes* mosquito. The Punjab Fisheries Department had stocked more than 100,000 fish in 107 different sites.

Biological Control of Dengue

During a meeting held on the subject of vector control, the Chief Minister Punjab desired for biological control of *Aedes* mosquito through introduction of predator fish in the water bodies of different cities of Punjab.

In this respect initial surveys were conducted for identification of potential water bodies. The basic objectives of the survey was to identify water bodies that could act as ideal habitat for both the fish and the *Aedes* mosquitoes. The survey was followed by the release of two species of fish namely the Talapia and Grass Carp. The impact of such biological control included the eradication of eggs and larvae of mosquito in ponds and ditches of water.

The Grass Carp consumes the ingrown aquatic vegetation, which otherwise serves to anchor larvae and mosquito. The departmental experts later introduced the Gambusia Affinis commonly known as mosquito fish in the various ponds of Lahore. The advantage of this species is that it has the ability to self breed 3-4 times in a season and matures in six to eight weeks. The downside however is that being an invasive species, it can affect the local fish culture . The Gambusia was cultured in the Uchali Complex of district Khushab and later transported to Lahore. Approximately 2,500 fish were released at different sites in the city.

The Fisheries Department not only introduced the fish in the affected areas, but it also monitored the areas on a continual basis to ensure the effectiveness of their biological control.

Policy Guidelines

The administrators of areas facing a risk of Dengue outbreak should create a similar biological control program. Fish such as Tilapia, Grass-Carp and Gambusia, feed on the larvae of *Aedes* Mosquitoes. These species should be cultured in a controlled environment and then introduced to ponds where *Aedes* mosquitoes can lay their eggs.

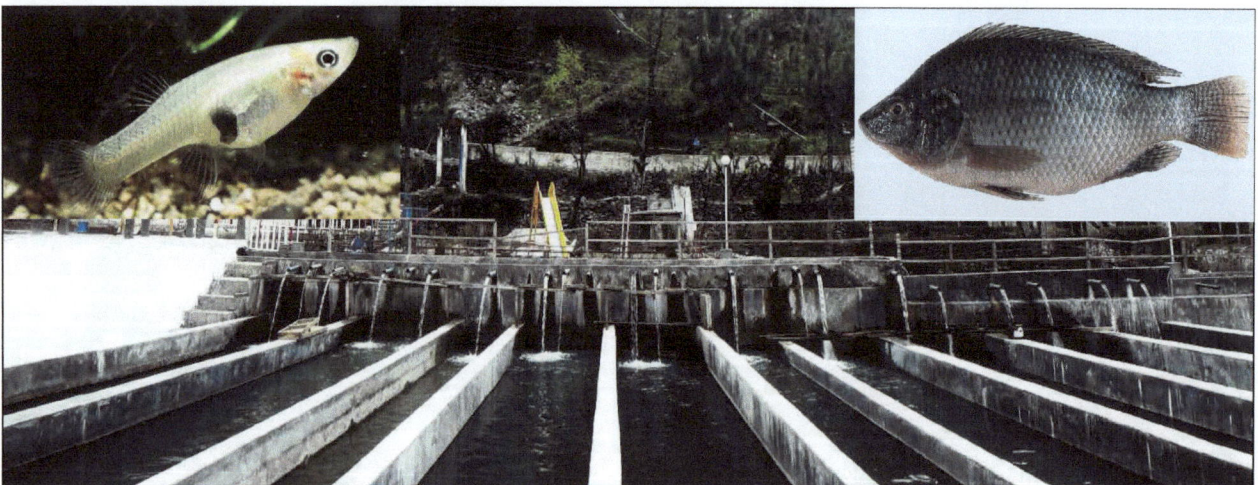

More than 100,000 Talapia & Grass Carp Fish were stocked and released   Fig. 47

Lahore Waste Management Company (LWMC) launched an aggressive campaign for cleanliness and removal of garbage. Garbage and debris provides a conducive and humid environment where small puddles of water can get accumulated. The proper disposal of garbage decreases the possibility of excessive breeding as it does not allow the creation of vector habitats among the urban refuse. Stagnant water in plastic cups or cardboard boxes can allow breeding if left unattended. The LWMC strove to eradicate the possibility of any such breeding by taking care of the garbage that the city generated.

LWMC undertook the following activities:

• Removal of the solid waste/garbage from open/vacant plots

• Removal of Dengue larvae hot spots that were identified by the entomological survey of the Agriculture Department

• Redressal of complaints that were collected through the Electronic Complaint Routing System (ECRS)

LWMC cleared two thousand vacant plots and removed approximately 131,000 tons of garbage including the Construction & Demolition (C&D) waste. This task was accomplished by hiring equipment and machinery from private contractors. Every day 4,000 tons of solid waste, in addition to the routine waste collection, was lifted, transported and dumped at waste disposal facilities in Lahore. The community was also encouraged to identify filthy plots and convey it to the LWMC for removal of garbage.

The problematic target areas in each Union Council (UC) were identified and special Group Activities were carried out on daily basis to resolve the cleanliness problems in identified areas. The objective of such group activities was to consolidate the resources and plan their utilization. The resources were pooled up and at least 20-50 additional sanitary workers were used to participate in each such activity. These workers contributed in street/road sweeping, waste collection and

transfer of the waste to containers that were transported to a disposal site using arm roll truck, open truck, master pickups, or front end loaders.

LWMC remained actively engaged in the removal of larvae hotspots identified by the Agriculture Department. LWMC addressed 128 such spots by cleaning those areas. A number of citizens utilized the ECRS to report the presence of garbage in the open area. LWMC responded to more than 800 calls and then called back the complainants to ensure their satisfaction with the service delivered.

In order to create an awareness about general cleanliness, LWMC launched an awareness campaign encouraging people to discourage the vector breeding by maintaining a state of cleanliness in their areas and by contacting LWMC for the removal of garbage from any open plots. The LWMC telephone Helpline 1139 was also communicated to the citizens of Lahore.

The Special Branch of the Punjab Police was assigned the task of monitoring the work done by LWMC. This branch identified 390 places, which were all eventually cleaned.

LWMC also sought to clear the back log of waste related concerns raised in the different UCs of Lahore. The department facilitated the field officers of different UCs by providing them with the adequate machinery.

LWMC cleaning team in action   *Fig. 48*

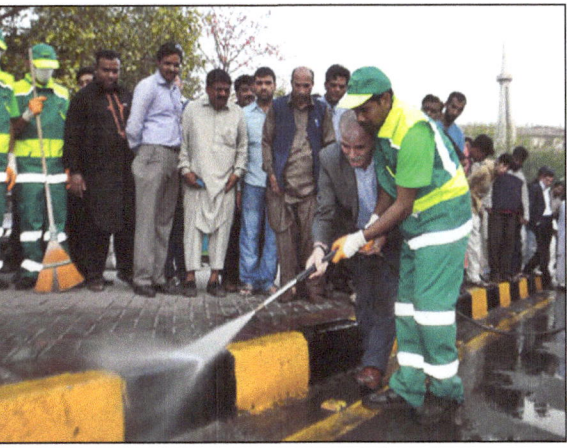

Local Government and Community Development (LG&CD) initiated a comprehensive fumigation and cleanliness drive at Graveyards across Lahore. The department conducted two rounds of fumigation at 275 out of 300 Graveyards of urban Lahore that are not located in private housing societies. Department's fumigation and cleanliness drive consisted of three essential actions to remove all possible habitats of *Aedes* mosquitoes:

- Fumigation
- Cleaning
- Grubbing

The department has placed a special emphasis on the 150 acre Miani Sahib Graveyard that contained 35 shrines, 75 water reservoirs and water tanks for ablution. Most of the water reservoirs were eliminated while the rest were disinfected by introducing lavicides. The shrines were disinfected by regular spraying of Internal Residual Spray while fogging was conducted in the entire Graveyard for three times.

The Government of Punjab passed a resolution to keep a strong check on the unwanted activity of rubber tyres. After the promulgation of the regulation against unwanted activity of tires, departments could take action against parties that refused to conform to such rules. The LG&CDdepartment confiscated 2,888 tyres and chopped them off.

LG&CD contributed to the public awareness campaign by distributing countless pamphlets and 800 CDs to people across the Punjab province. The department also organized seminars with trade unions, voluntary organizations and NGOs.

The LG&CD Department identified 54 Graveyards for infrastructure improvement which were improved by cleaning pathways and Wazu-Gahs (Ablution Locations)

Fumigation of Graveyards in Lahore City

The fumigation of graveyards was spearheaded by the LG&CD Department. However it did entail the cooperation of the Religious Affairs Department, Cantonment Board, and Graveyard Committees. Miani Sahib Graveyard is the largest in Lahore spanning a vast area of 150 acres. This vast Graveyard was severly infected with larvae before the intevention. The Grave-diggers had made more than 70 water-pits to store the water that they needed to soften the soil before digging. Almost all of those water pits were infected with larvae. The area around this graveyard had a large number of Dengue patients due to this very reason. The Miani Sahib Graveyard falls in the Union Council (UC) of Mozang. More than 200 patients had been reported from Mozang in about two months. In most of the other UCs of Lahore, the number of patients was less than 50. Comparatively speaking, Mozang was one of the worst affected areas of Lahore and the primary reason behind the outbreak was the availability of favorable breeding sites for *Aedes* mosquitoes in the Miani Sahib graveyard. The LG&CD Department responded to this crisis by conducting a three day long fumigation in the Miani Sahib Graveyard.

Fumigation process in Miani Sahib *Fig. 49*

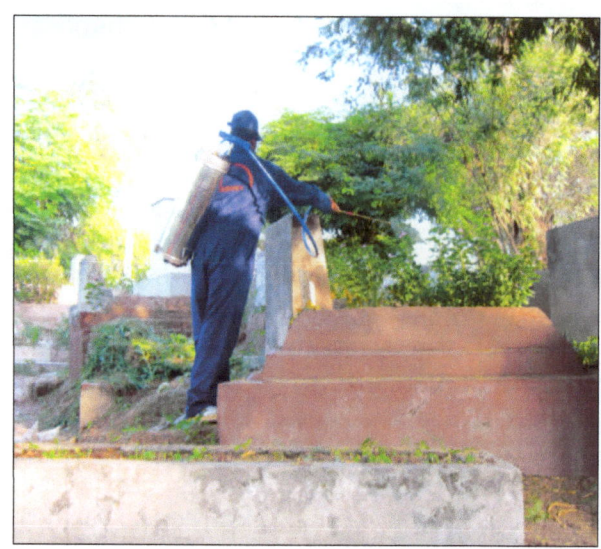

Punjab Information Technology Board (PITB) setup an Electronic Complaint Routing System (ECRS) that received more than a hundred thousand Dengue related complaints and routed them to the concerned departments. During the outbreak, hundreds of thousands of Lahore's citizens called on the toll free telephone number 0800-99000 to report issues such as the short comings in the health services, and identification of ideal breeding spots for the *Aedes* mosquitoes. The complaints received by the PITB were then categorized and delivered to the department best suited to address them. PITB hired 150 doctors to respond to citizen's concerns regarding the fever. These 150 doctors operated the call centre in three shifts around the clock. PITB received about 5,000 calls each day when the epidemic out-break was at its peak.

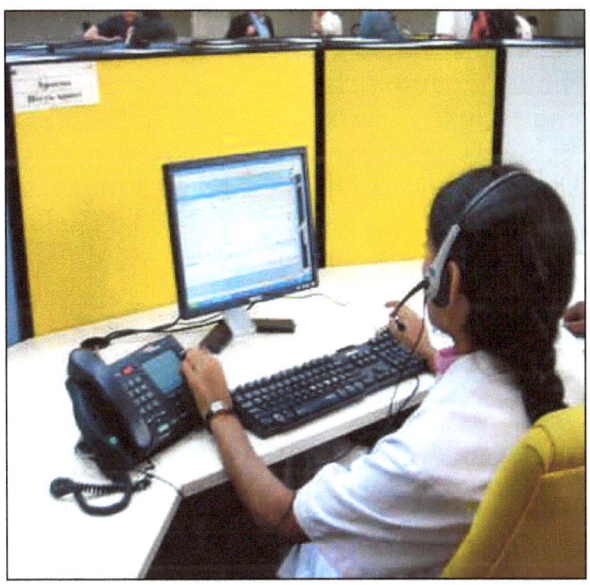

PITB worker responding a call   *Fig. 50*

Sample template of the types of complaints   *Table: 15*

No.	Issue	Complaints	Routed to Department
1	Cleanliness	43	LWMC
2	Fog Spray	263	TMA
3	IRS	1,784	TMA
4	Government Hospital Charging	3	DG Health
5	Government Hospital	13	DG Health
6	Private Hospital Overcharging	5	CDGL Health
7	Private Lab Overcharging	6	CDGL Health
8	Sewerage Blockage	10	WASA
9	Water Supply	1	WASA
10	Ponding	30	WASA
11	School Spray	3	Secy. Schools
12	Chemical Control	96	TMA
13	Over Charging Medicine	1	DG Health
14	Others	-	DG Health
	Total	**2,258**	

The Higher Education Department conducted a mass awareness campaign by mobilizing the college and university students. The department distributed hundreds of thousands of pamphlets, created a documentary and setup road-side camps with the help of students. Students were provided with Dengue prevention checklists so that they could convince other members of their families to prevent their homes from the influx of Dengue.

Launching Students for Social Action

The Higher Education Department's awareness campaign emphasized general cleanliness, eradication of potential breeding spots and fumigation of current vector habitats. The main objective of the exercise was to build the capacity of the residents of Lahore to support the vector control. The department setup 387 road-side camps at 39 different spots which distributed 700,000 pamphlets. The mass awareness campaign urged the residents of Lahore to share the responsibility and play their own role in eradicating mosquitoe breeding areas in their houses and work places.

Capacity Building

The Higher Education Department conducted 110 workshops and seminars in 55 different educational institutions of Lahore (see table 16). Two workshops were held in every college or higher secondary school. The workshops constituted of a documentary highlighting the identification of *Aedes* mosquitoes, and methods of eradicating its habitats. The documentary was usually followed by a motivational address by experts and an interactive session. The workshops concluded by breaking the students into smaller groups to get them involved in informative exercises.

Post-workshop Activities

Students were provided with Dengue prevention checklists that they took to their homes. These checklists required the students to conform to certain household practices of mechanical control. These students were also required to submit the filled checklists back to their teachers. The teachers then conducted a brief workshop on the findings of the checklists returned to them. Final certificates were also distributed to the best participants of the awareness exercise.

Student mobilization for Dengue awareness   *Fig. 51*

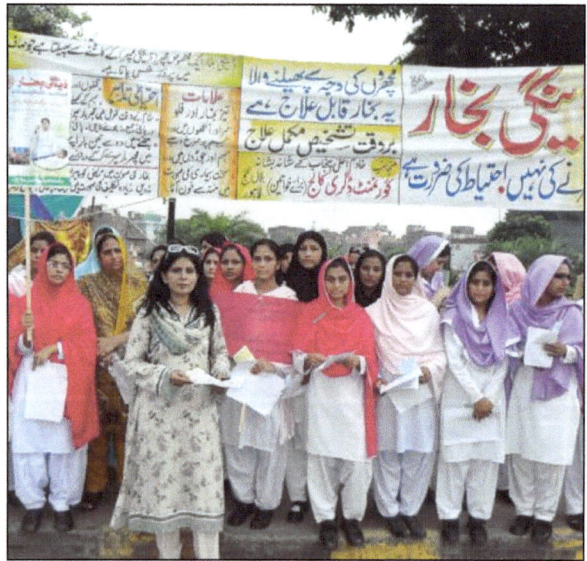
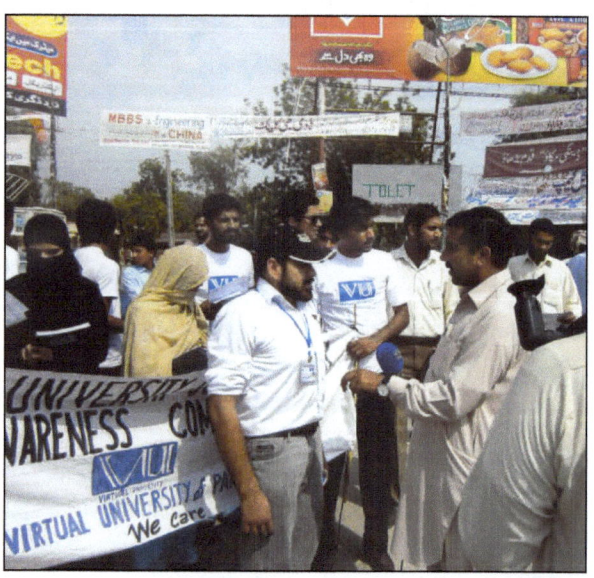

List of awareness workshops at major colleges
Table: 16

No.	Name of the College	1st. Seminar/ Workshop	2nd. Workshop	Cleanliness Week
1	Govt. Islamia College (W) Cooper Road	26th Sep. 11	10th Oct.11	3rd Oct. to 08th Oct. 11
2	Govt. M.A.O. College Lahore	26th Sep.11	10th Oct.11	3rd Oct. to 08th Oct. 11
3	Govt. Girls H.S.S. Dev Smaj Road	26th Sep.11	10th Oct.11	3rd Oct. to 08th Oct. 11
4	Govt. Post Graduate College	27th Sep.11	11th Oct. 11	3rd Oct. to 08th Oct.11
5	Govt. Islamia College Civil Lines	27th Sep.11	11th Oct. 11	3rd Oct. to 08th Oct. 11
6	Govt. College for Women Gulberg	28th Sep.11	12th Oct. 11	3rd Oct. to 08th Oct. 11
7	Govt. College Of Science Wahdat Road	28th Sep.11	12th Oct. 11	3rd Oct. to 08th Oct. 11
8	Govt. Girls H.S.S. Allama Iqbal Town	28th Sep.11	12th Oct. 11	3rd Oct. to 08th Oct. 11
9	Govt. College of Home Economics	29th Sep. 11	13th Oct. 11	3rd Oct. to 08th Oct. 11
10	Govt. College Township	29th Sep. 11	13th Oct. 11	3rd Oct. to 08th Oct. 11
11	Govt. H.S.S. for Boys, Green Town	29th Sep. 11	13th Oct. 11	3rd Oct. to 08th Oct. 11
12	Govt. College for Women Wahdat Colony	30th Sep. 11	14th Oct.11	3rd Oct. to 08th Oct.11
13	Govt. Jinnah Degree College (W) Mozang	30th Sep. 11	14th Oct.11	3rd Oct. to 08th Oct. 11
14	Govt. College (Boys), Model Town	01st Oct. 11	15th Oct.11	10th Oct. to 15th Oct. 11
15	Govt. College (W) E-block Model Town	01st Oct. 11	15th Oct.11	10th Oct. to 15th Oct.11
16	Govt. Girls H.S.S. Awan Town	01st Oct. 11	15th Oct.11	10th Oct. to 15th Oct. 11
17	Govt. Girls H.S.S. Shahdara	3rd Oct. 11	17th Oct.11	10th Oct. to 15th Oct. 11

Policy Guidelines:

The administrators should mobilize the youth to raise awareness on means and methods through which the residents of their area can prevent themselves from Dengue fever. College and University students are willing contributors to the vector control efforts. They can assist in the distribution of leaflets, and conduction of seminars on Dengue prevention. They can also convince people in their neighborhoods to refrain from piling debris that can act as habitat for *Aedes* Mosquitoes.

The administration should also initiate a school cleanliness drive in which the schools should be cleaned, fumigated and inspected. Spraying machines and medicines should be provided to schools and colleges. Teachers should be instructed on the Dengue prevention strategies as well as the symptoms that they might observe in their students.

The various activities of awareness campaigns utilizing school resources and students may be documented using the sample template in table 17.

Sample template for documentation of awareness campaigns
Table: 17

No.	Name of College	Distribution of Pamphlets	Workshop	Seminar	Cleanliness Week

Perhaps the largest department of Punjab is the School Education Department, which looks after 1.45 million students in district Lahore alone (see table 18). It conducted a comprehensive chemical control in all of the government and private schools. Two rounds of Internal Residual Spray were conducted in all government schools. A cleanliness drive was initiated in all school premises. Unserviceable furniture, broken flower pots and debris were removed. The sewerage system, water taps and washrooms were cleaned and maintained. Overgrown grass and hedges were trimmed to avoid any unidentified accumulation of water. Stagnant water on the rooftops of schools was drained.

The School Education Department closed the schools for 10 working days when the epidemic outbreak had reached its peak. The transfer of vector-borne virus from one person to another was taking place on a large scale putting the school students at a high risk of Dengue fever at that time. Hence closure of schools was deemed essential to save the lives of school going children. During those ten days, the school premises were fumigated and cleaned of all potential habitats of *Aedes* mosquitoes. School students were educated on Dengue and its symptoms.

The morning assemblies and evening games were suspended and students were encouraged to wear full sleeve shirts, trousers and close shoes with socks. The department also printed advertisements in the newspapers, which sought the parents' attention to prevent their school going children from exposure to *Aedes* mosquitoes.

Awareness Campaign

The School Education Department conducted a mass awareness campaign to orient teachers, students and parents about the prevention and control of Dengue fever. The department mobilized a number of scouts for the execution of this campaign. The teachers were equipped with the required material to conduct seminars. Special posters were affixed in schools and 1.3 million leaflets were distributed to the general public and students. Students were also equipped with information material that they could take to their homes.

The department incorporated certain Dengue related information in the school curriculum as well. A zero period on methods of preventing the Dengue fever was held at various schools of Lahore.

The World Health Organization (WHO) designed a booklet for teachers and students. The booklets, in Urdu language, articulated the methods of lowering the risk of Malaria and Dengue fever (Figure 51). The School Education Department distributed the book to over 50,000 persons.

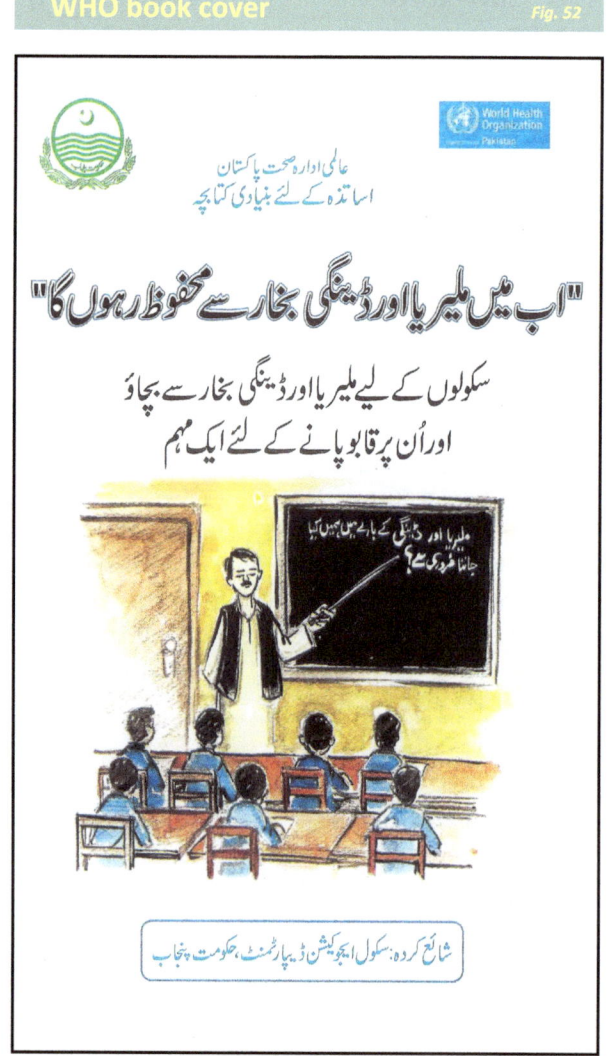

WHO book cover *Fig. 52*

Schools in District Lahore

Table: 18

No.	Category	Schools	Students
1	Government Sector Schools	1,250	581,000
2	Private Sector Schools	4,605	870,000
	Total:	5,855	1,451,000

Students partcipating in anti-Dengue awareness campaigns

Fig. 53

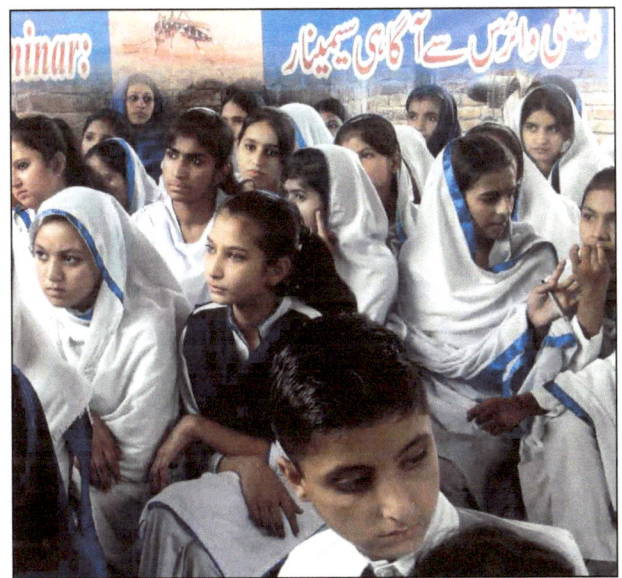
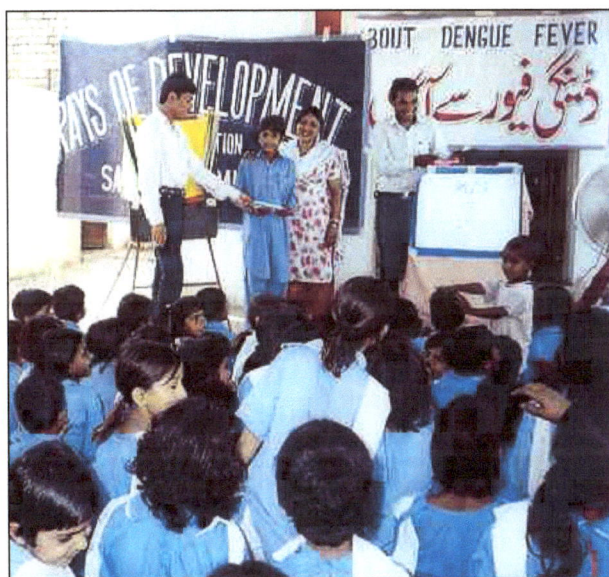
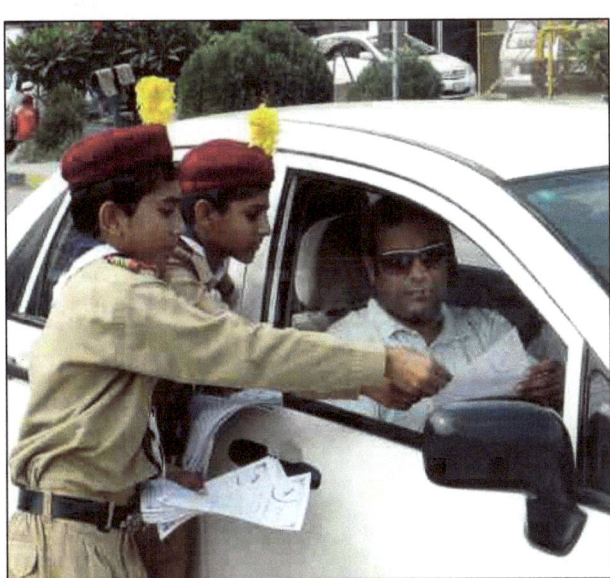
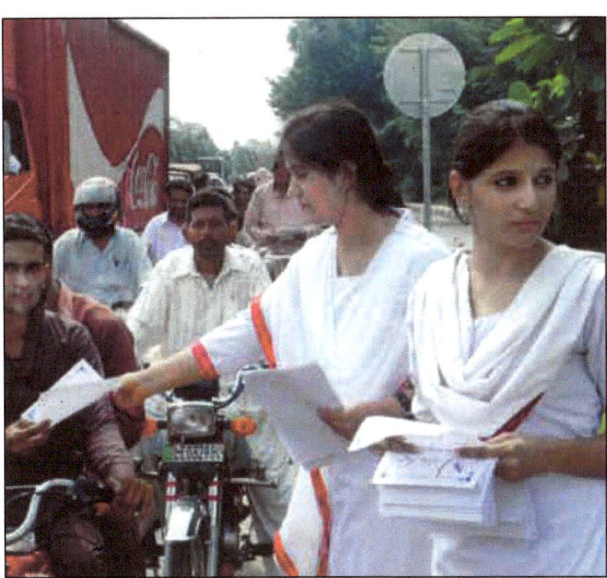

The Social Welfare Department acts as an intermediary between the government machinery and Non-Governmental Organizations (NGOs) for better utilization of the cumulative resources. It coordinated with the NGOs to provide healthcare services to a number of patients with Dengue related symptoms. The hospitals and trusts operated by NGOs were used to fill whatever gap was left between the resources at government's disposal and the resources that were required in the face of the rising number of patients. NGOs were encouraged to setup medical camps that could act as referral points. The Social Welfare Department mobilized the NGOs to supplement the vector control efforts of other governmental departments. Tables 19-21 give details of some such facilities along with their Dengue beds, Labs and patient details.

The department also mobilized teams of community volunteers in 150 Union Councils for dissemination of awareness related material. The department held a convention of NGOs at Al-Hamra Hall, Lahore, and five seminars at different towns of Lahore. The department oversaw the operations of 75 awareness camps setup by the NGOs and the deployment of 34 NGO staff members at 17 different diagnostic centers setup by the Health Department.

Sample template of Dengue related work undertaken by NGO's

Table: 19

No.	Name of the NGO	Total Beds	Beds for Dengue Patients	OPD	Lab
1	Ch Rehmat Memorial Hospital	300	80	400	IGM, IGG, CBC (Free)
2	Al-Ehsan Hospital	65	62	100	CBC (Free)
3	Surraya Azeem Hospital	350	60	100	CBC (Rs 50)
4	Fatima Memorial Hospital	540	60	200	CBC (Free)
5	Hijaz Hospital, Gulberg	100	35	300	IGM, IGG, CBC (Subsidized)
6	Mumtaz Bakhtawar, Raiwind Road	100	30	200	CBC (Free)
7	Mumtaz Bakhtawar, Wahdat Road	80	30	200	CBC (Free)
8	Mansoora Hospital	150	30	200	CBC (Rs 50)
9	Society Hospital	30	13	100	CBC (Free)
10	Zainab Hospital, Gulberg	20	10	50	CBC (Free)
11	Mukhtaran Rafique Hospital	10	05	50	CBC (Free)
	Total	**1,745**	**415**	**1,900**	

Policy Guidelines

The administrators should mobilize the NGOs to provide healthcare services to patients with Dengue related symptoms. The hospitals and trusts operated by NGOs should also be engaged to ensure supplementary services in case the number of patients exceeds at a rapid pace. NGOs should be encouraged to setup medical camps in worst affected areas and provide relief to families that have been worst affected by this fever.

Sample template of laboratory resources available at NGO operated hospitals — Table: 20

No.	Name of the NGO	Commitment
1	Sundas Foundation	IGG, IGM, CBC *(Free, subject to availability of test kits)*
2	Al-Ehsan Hospital	Printing of awareness material
3	Mansoora Hospital	Printing of awareness material
4	Nagina Foundation	Arrangement of spray, Blood donation, free medicine
5	Anti-Narcotics Youth Force	Medical Camps

Sample template of patients treated at various NGO operated hospitals (15th Oct. 2011) — Table: 21

No.	Name of Hospital	Total Beds	Beds reserved for Dengue	Patients Investigated	Suspected/ Confirmed	Total admitted	Total discharged	Admitted
1	Mumtaz Bakhtawar Raiwind Road	100	30	110	17	35	18	17
2	Mumtaz Bakhtawar Wahdat Road	80	60	92	--	12	7	5
3	Mansoora Multan Road	150	30	149	1	31	2	29
4	Ch.Rehmat Ali Trust Hospital	300	80	170	--	55	11	44
5	Mukhtaran Rafiq	10	10	132	7	7	4	3
6	Al-Ehsan Eye	65	62	230	24	24	18	6
7	Society Hospital	30	13	96	1	1	1	-
8	Hijaz Hospital	100	35	144	--	4	4	0
9	Zanbia Hospital	20	10	80	5	-	-	-
10	Surraya Azeem	350	60	254	10	34	4	30
11	Fatima Memorial	540	60	366	5	52	5	47
	Total	**1,745**	**440**	**1,823**	**70**	**178**	**74**	**104**

The Transport Department took preventive measures at bus terminals/wagon stands, bus depots and tyre shops. Seven special squads were formed to carry out the inspection of bus terminals on a daily basis. The seven squads were supported with ten teams of the Environment Department for actions against the tyre shops violating government's regulations for tyre management. Tyres lying in the open were removed, treated properly and stored under sheds. The inspection teams ensured that there was no stagnant water in the premises of bus terminals. Special attention was paid to eradicate any puddles near the water dispensers, bathrooms and airconditioning units that condense water in pots or other utensils. All buses departing Lahore were sprayed 30 minutes before the boarding of passengers. Banners promoting personal Dengue prevention were displayed at all bus terminals for awareness of commuters as well as transporters. Pamphlets and leaflets on Dengue control were also distributed among commuters by the transporters themselves. The Transport Department held regular meetings with the transporters to encourage them to keep the waiting areas, vehicles and allied places free of garbage, stagnant water and open tyre stocks.

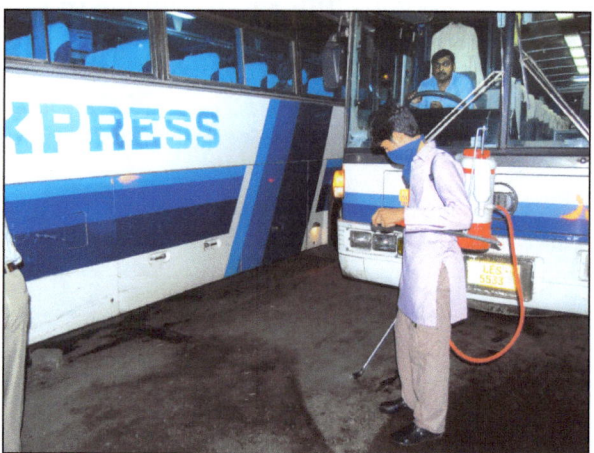
Dengue control spray at Bus Terminals   Fig. 54

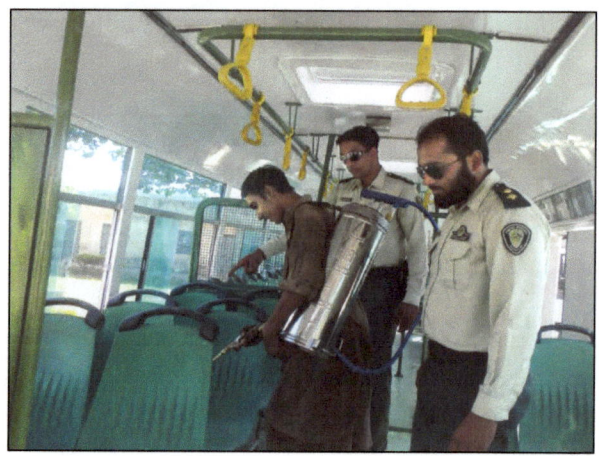

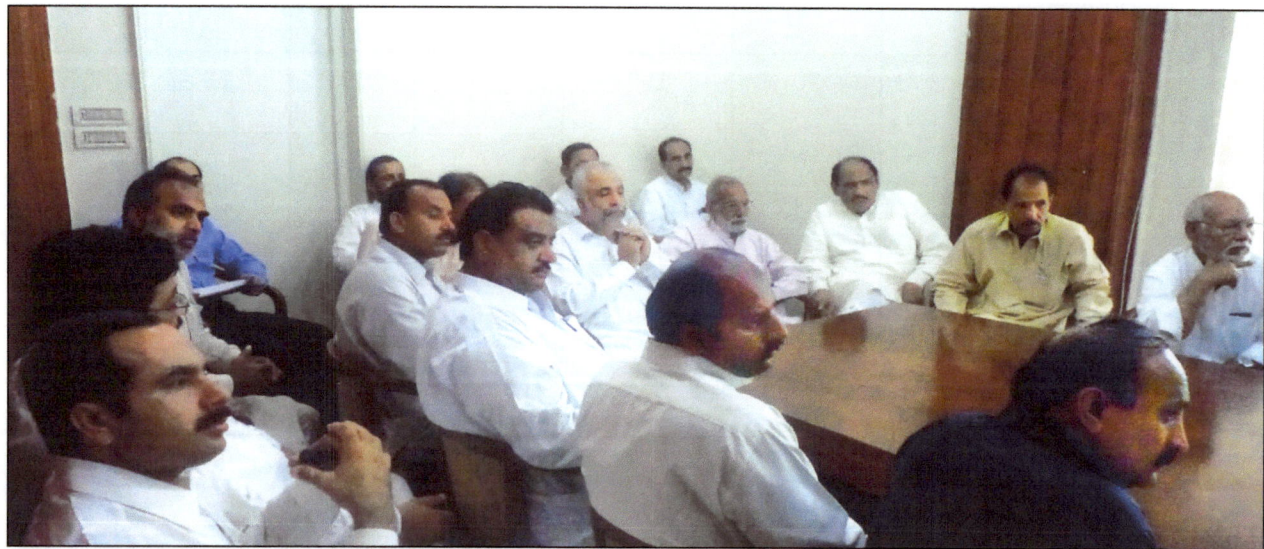
Transporters meet to combat Dengue at Bus Terminals   Fig. 55

The Water and Sanitation Agency (WASA) recieved and responded to complaints regarding the accumulation of unwanted water and resolved almost all of the dewatering related complaints. WASA had maintained an optimum discharge rate in all water supply and sewerage channels of Lahore, to ensure that all sewerage is drained.

Excess in the discharge rate can overflow the water creating ideal breeding sites for the *Aedes* mosquitoes. The residents of Lahore utilized the Electronic Complaint Routing System (ECRS) to communicate complaint locations. WASA then responded by engaging pumps, muck suckers and dewatering sets to clear the stagnant water (Table 22).

Complaints received and Dewatering operations conducted at various areas on 1st Oct 2011 *Table: 22*

No.	O&M Towns	Water Supply		Sewerage	
		Received	Attended	Received	Attended
1	Ravi Town	23	21	95	91
2	Gunj Baksh Town	18	18	115	109
3	Nishtar Town	8	7	42	37
4	Shalimar Town	8	5	27	23
5	Iqbal Town	11	10	71	60
6	Complaint Monitoring Cell	26	8	25	2
	Total	94	69	375	322

No.	Location		Machinery
	RAVI TOWN		
1	Kala Khatai Road	Dewatering Sets	Intermediate Pumping
2	Abbas Nagar Degree College		
3	Saeed Park Army Ground		In Operation
4	Ravi Clifton Near Saleem Garden		
5	Baigum Bagh Tiearh		
6	Chatta Park F/Abad	Muck Sucker Dewatering Sets	
7	Pindi Das Road F/Abad		
8	Gulshan-e-Hayat Park		
9	Badshah Road Block-A-II China Scheme		
10	Shaheen Park, Bhaghatpura		
11	590 A/2, China Scheme		Clear
12	Khuda Buksh, Baghatpura		In Operation
13	Yousuf Park	Dewatering Sets	In Operation
	GUNJ BUKSH TOWN		
14	Ghulam Hussain Colony	Dewatering Sets	In Operation
	ALLAMA IQBAL TOWN		
15	Open Plot Behind Mian Plaza	Dewatering Sets	In Operation
16	N-Block Pond Johar Town		
17	H-3 Block, Johar Town		
18	Madni Masjid, Azam Garden		

The province of Punjab is divided into nine Divisions (Figure 55), which are further divided into 36 Districts. Lahore is one of the nine Divisions of Punjab and within this Division, the Disctrict of Lahore is the area that this book has highlighted uptill this point. Apart from the Lahore District, the Division of Lahore is composed of three other districts namely Nankana Sahib, Sheikhupura and Kasur. These neighboring districts of Lahore were also affected by the epidemic outbreak but the number of patients identified in these areas was not as high as that of Faisalabad and Rawalpindi Districts. Thousands of people commute between these three cities on a daily basis. This inter-city travelling is largely attributed to the proliferation of Lahore's Dengue fever to other major cities.

The following section discusses the Dengue control efforts of Faisalabad Division as an example. All other Divisions took similar measures. Monthly meetings of all nine Divisional Commissioners were regularly conducted by the Chief Minister.

Faisalabad Division is further divided into the Districts of Faisalabad, Jhang, Chiniot, and Toba Tek Singh. Faisalabad Division initiated vector control in the same fashion as Lahore. Fogging was conducted in the open, Internal Residual Spray was conducted indoors and larviciding was conducted in water ponds that had to be retained. Distict wise details of vector control are given in table 23 where as details of Awareness Campaign material are given in table 24.

Nine Divisions of Punjab Province *Fig. 56*

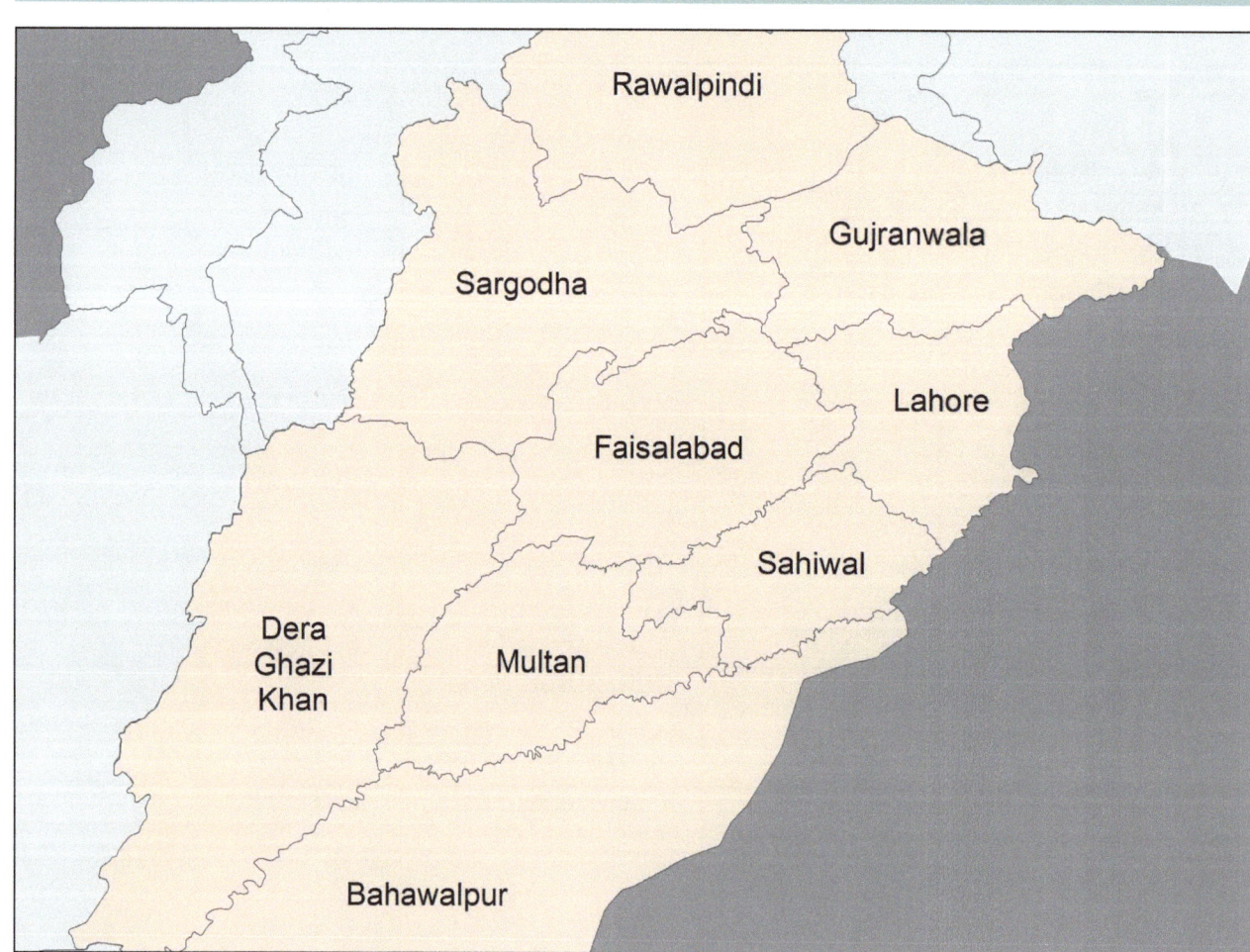

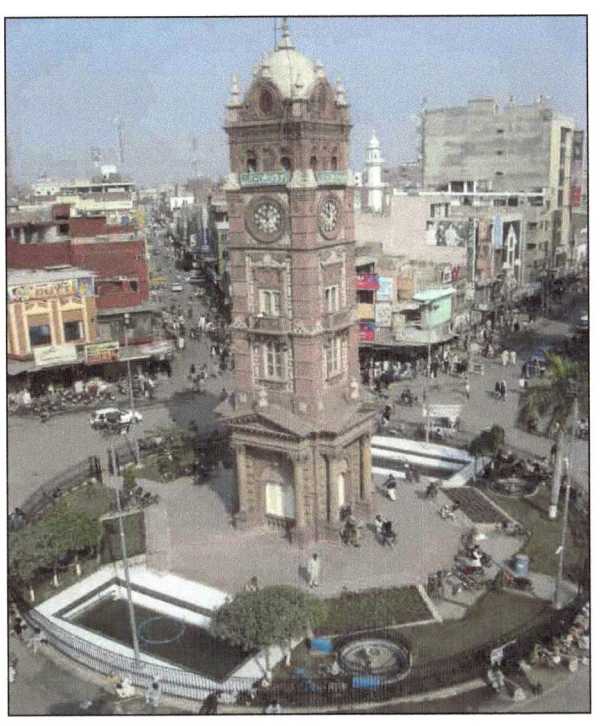

Faisalabad City   Fig. 57

The administrators of the Faisalabad Division conducted fogging in all of its Districts. Special emphasis was given to parks, colleges, and hospitals. The District Coordination Officers convened daily meetings at their offices to plan the Dengue control efforts. The administrators of the Faisalabad Division also planned and executed a comprehensive awareness campaign to obtain citizen's support in Dengue control.

Thousands of pamphlets were distributed and numerours awareness sessions were held at Schools and Townhalls. Separate counters and isolation wards were established for Dengue patients in the hospitals. The ELISA test for confirmation of Dengue fever was established as a free service.

Hematology Analyzers were made available at all hospitals. Platelets Kits were made available for free and the testing service for platelet count was established at all the Rural Health Centers (RHCs)

Sample template of Chemical Control in Faisalabad Division — Table: 23

No.	Description	Faisalabad	Jhang	T.T. Singh	Chiniot
1	Total UC's	113	18	16	12
2	Fogging Completed	113	18	16	12
3	Fogging Repeated	96	18	16	12
4	Parks Sprayed	289	20	300	10
5	Hospitals Sprayed	20	11	50	06
6	Colleges / Schools Sprayed	95	83	500	75
7	Nomad Camps	438	09	557	80
8	Green Belts	25	05	55	03
Larvicidal Operation					
1	Ponds covered	1846	67	800	80
2	UC's Completed	113	18	16	12

Sample template of Awareness Material distributed in Faisalabad division *Table: 24*

No.	Description	Faisalabad	Jhang	T.T. Singh	Chiniot
1	Distribution of pamphlets / leaflets	180,000	110,000	66,000	4,300
2	Holding of Health Education Sessions in 340 Educational Institutions.	148	5,500	27	
3	School teachers trained for public awareness	2,400	115	1,500	150
4	Medical students mobilized for public awareness campaign	All students	08	N/A	N/A
5	NGO's involved in monitoring Dengue activities and in public awareness campaign	13	06	05	05
6	Involvement of print / electronic media	Yes	Yes	News Papers	Yes
7	Holding of Seminars	148	97	04	
8	Displaying of Banners / Posters at prominent places including Rural Areas	Banners 480, Posters 15,000	Banners 537, Charts 500	500	Banners 365, Posters 3,000
9	Awareness Walks arranged by NGO's & Government	12	06	05	05
10	Seminars conducted on facility of testing	15	05	-	04
11	CDs regarding awareness shown in all Town Halls	Yes	Yes	04	Yes
12	CDs have been distributed to all the Schools	Yes	Yes	110	Yes
13	Free availability of test ensured at Govt. Hospitals and Rs. 90/- at all the Private Labs.	Yes	Yes	Yes	Yes

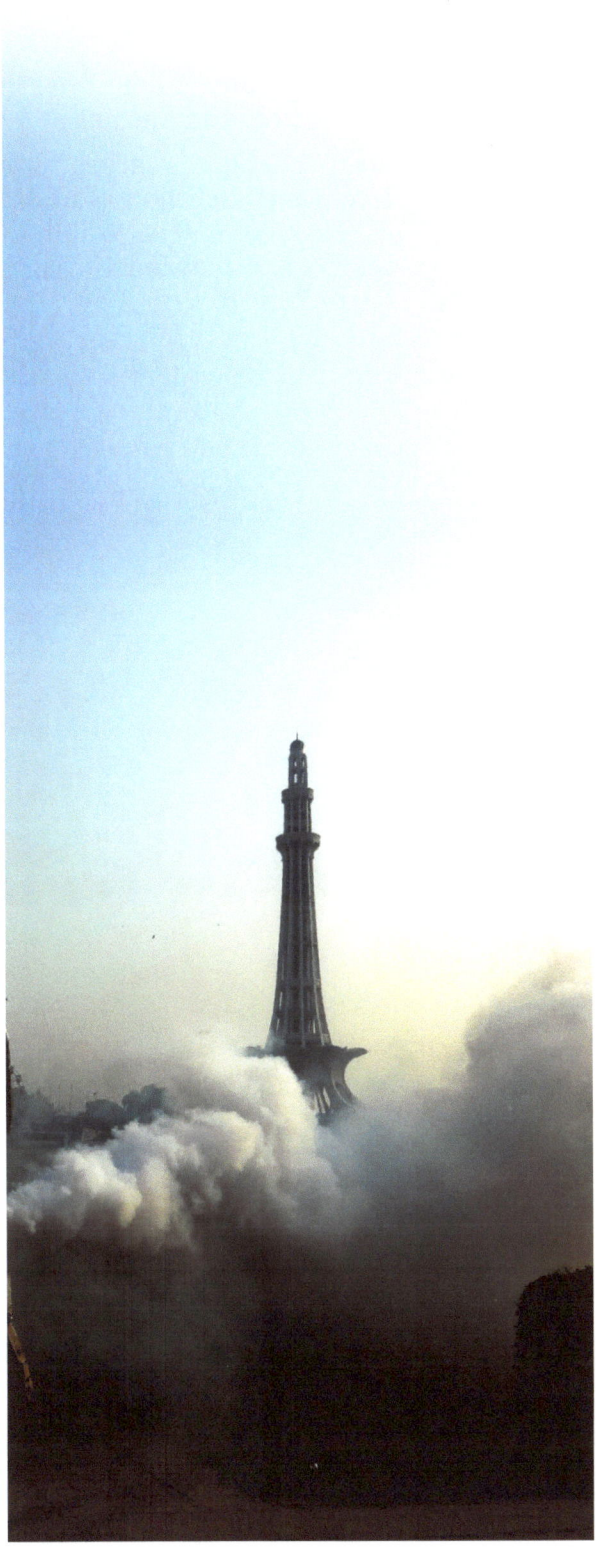

Although Punjab saw a massive Dengue outbreak in the year 2011, it would have been substantially worse had the government not responded in a timely and forceful manner.

Pakistan has a tropical climate conducive to the rapid breeding of mosquitoes. An integrated vector control program would not deliver the desired results unless the masses were engaged in a collaborative effort to eliminate this epidemic.

This book on Dengue prevention and control not only sheds light on the immediate measures that the administration should take to eradicate the source of this disease but also talks about awareness campaigns that should be conducted by engaging and mobilizing students and other relevant stakeholders.

All Governmental Departments have to contribute to the integrated vector control program. It is only with the cooperation of all stakeholders that an administrator can ensure all citizens of Pakistan a healthier and prosperous future. This book provides policy guidelines for the adminstrators of various govenment departments to combat Dengue in their respective fields.

It is hoped this text is circulated in libraries as a primary and original data-cum-narrative for reference in future research in fields of Public Health, Public Administration and Clinical studies.

Khalid Sherdil

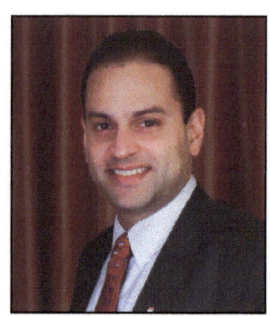

As Director General for the Provincial Disaster Management Authority, Punjab, Khalid Sherdil worked on Pakistan's largest ever disaster, the Super Floods of 2010.

Khalid has worked on six major disasters, including the Turkish Earthquake, Sindh Floods 2011 and Sialkot Tornado. Besides Dengue, Khalid has also written a technical report for Ontario Government on West Nile virus, another mosquito vector epidemic. He was also the Project Director of the Model Villages Project ($20 million), in which 22 villages equipped with schools, technical training centers, dispensaries, parks, solar electricity, bio-gas, etc., were constructed all over Punjab's Flood areas. He also led the project for disbursement of flood-damage compensation ($ 325 million in form of debit cards) to over 1 million flood-affected families of Punjab. He is a member of Pakistan's Core Committee for Environment and Climate Change, and has represented the country at COP 16 Cancun, Mexico.

Khalid has served as the Deputy Secretary for Information Technology Department, and for Agriculture Department, Government of the Punjab. His interest in Agriculture arises from his family farm where he cultivates wheat & rice in addition to Bio-Fuels. Earlier, he served as Assistant Commissioner of Murree and Lahore Cantt.

Khalid has Masters and Bachelors degrees in Computer Science (McGill University, Canada and Washington University, USA), and a Liberal Arts Bachelors in Physics (College of Wooster, USA). He is also an Electrical Engineer (Washington University). He is currently obtaining a Doctoral degree in Computer and Environmental Science at the Western University, Canada. His research interests are in Early Warning in Complex Adaptive Systems by Multi-Agent-SWARMS in Cloud Computing; and in applications of technology to environmental & sustainable development.

Khalid has twelve research publications in International Conferences and Journals.

Khalid also runs Pakistan's largest arts website ArtsPak.com and is a Fellow of LEAD International UK. He is currently also authoring a photographic book on the Model Villages and the Rural life of Punjab.

Faran Naru

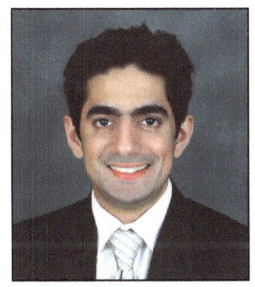

Faran Naru works as a Policy Advisor at PD-MA. Apart from the epidemic research, he also works on contingency planning of the provincial government.

Faran is a development consultant by profession and has provided his services to various international organizations and NGOs. Faran conceived, built and operated Lahore's first Bio-diesel factory that recycles used vegetable oil into a perfect substitute of diesel fuel. He obtained his Masters degree in Public Policy from Brown University and studied the role of religion in politics at Harvard University. Faran studied in Ivy League institutions as a Fulbright Scholar and upon the completion of his academic program, he returned to Pakistan to help the Government with the epidemic that threatened a large population of his native city.

Faran's epidemic research identified the source of this disease by pointing out that the vector colonies had originally thrived in the Parks and Graveyards of Lahore. Faran is well trained in Geographic Information Systems (GIS) and has frequently used GIS to back his policy recommendations with empirical evidence. Faran is also credited with the development of Punjab's Disaster Response Plan that articulates the procedures that would be adopted by all government departments, in case the nation faces a natural emergency.

Faran has worked with various international organizations such as UNDP, World Bank, Asian Development Bank, and UNICEF. He is also an agricultural specialist and is currently working on the development of an innovative Center Pivot irrigation system.

Ahmad Rajwana

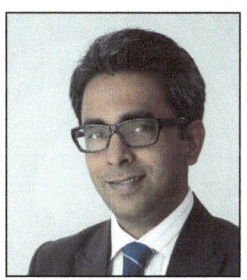

Ahmad Rajwana is currently Deputy Secretary to the Chief Minister, Punjab. He contributed to the vector control while working as the Director Operations at the Provincial Disaster Management Authority, Punjab.

He was appointed as a Director due to his formidable experience in disaster management. As the Chief Coordinator for Internally Displaced Persons of Malakand in Swabi, he streamlined the relief operations by devising an information system that documented over a million migrants. Maintaining a record of the mass movement allowed him to improve their shaken lives through special initiatives like subsistence through vocational training model, children play areas, psycho-social engagement and mobile health units.

In a subsequent assignment in post conflict Swat, he rehabilitated the agrarian economy and raised a new sub-division, Barikot. Ahmed is trained in Trade and Economic Development from Pakistan Institute of Trade Development and from London School of Economics.

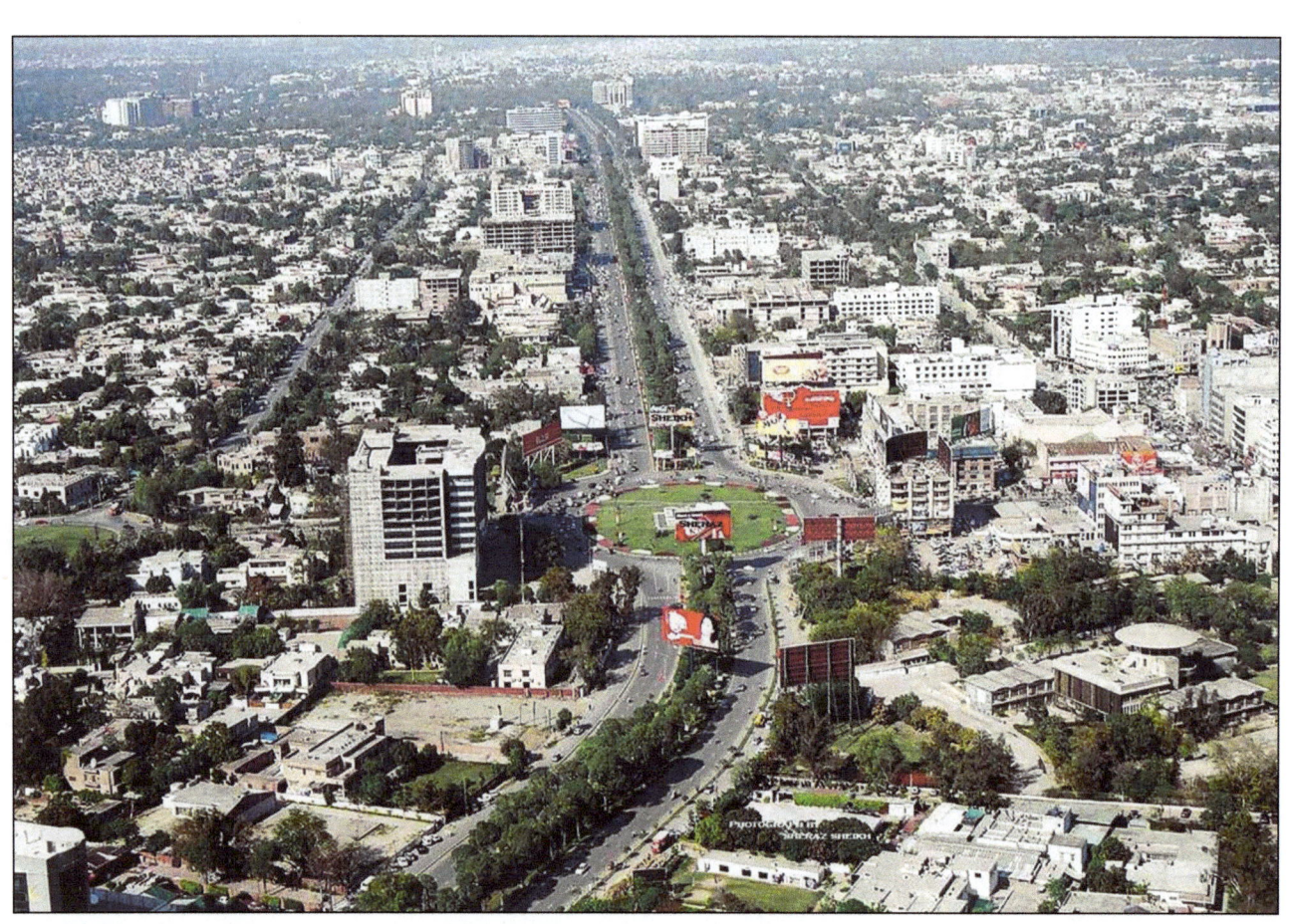

Aerial view of Liberty and its adjacent area (Gulberg Town) Lahore